PRIME FOR LIFE

PRIME FOR LIFE
FUNCTIONAL FITNESS FOR AGELESS LIVING

RANDY RAUGH, MPT

THE PROGRAM USED AT CANYON RANCH

RODALE

© 2009 by Randy Raugh

Rodale books may be purchased for business or promotional use or for special sales. For information, please write to:
Special Markets Department, Rodale Inc., 733 Third Avenue, New York, NY 10017

Printed in the United States of America
Rodale Inc. makes every effort to use acid-free ♾, recycled paper ♻.

Photographs by Mitch Mandel/Rodale Images
Illustrations by Karen Kuchar
Book design by Carol Angstadt

Library of Congress Cataloging-in-Publication Data

Raugh, Randy.
     Prime for life : functional fitness for ageless living / by Randy Raugh.
          p.   cm.
     Includes index.
     ISBN-13 978–1–59486–829–0 hardcover
     ISBN-10 1–59486–829–8 hardcover
     1. Physical fitness.   2. Exercise.   3. Joints.   I. Title.
     RA781.R295   2009
     613.7—dc22   2009009416

Distributed to the trade by Macmillan

2   4   6   8   10   9   7   5   3   1   hardcover

We inspire and enable people to improve their lives and the world around them
For more of our products visit **rodalestore.com** or call 800-848-4735

To my Lynne and Tyler,
without whom this wouldn't be.

"People usually consider walking on water or on thin air a miracle. But I think the real miracle is not to walk on either water or thin air, but to walk on earth."

—*Thich Nhat Hanh*

CONTENTS

AUTHOR'S NOTE

The Santa Catalina Mountains rise above Arizona like a blessing. Cradled in their shadows, heated by southwest sunshine, and fed by small streams that plummet from their slopes is Canyon Ranch, the world-renowned wellness and health center.

Each year, hundreds of people make the decision to leave the routines and restrictions of their daily lives and come to Canyon Ranch for a life-changing week. Within that short time, our guests reconnect with their bodies, their minds, and their hearts. They also reconnect with the natural world and their place in it as living, breathing—and moving—creatures.

My role as the fitness director of the Life Enhancement Program is to help people of all ages, and with all ranges of fitness levels, understand how movement and activity will not only bring them joy and excitement but will also protect them from disease, obesity, and the negative aspects of aging. And what do I mean by "movement and activity"? Just that—anything at all that keeps the body in motion, from carrying out the most subtle and mundane tasks to competing in elite sports.

People come to Canyon Ranch wanting to change. They want their lives to be better, richer, deeper, and more meaningful. And they want to engage in life with as much vigor and energy as possible. They know that at Canyon Ranch they will work with the most professional of instructors, practitioners, and health specialists—people who are on the cutting edge of the most recent developments in health care, physical therapy, nutrition, and exercise physiology.

Our team represents a philosophy of wellness that is both holistic and practical, spiritual and physically grounded. My role as a physical therapist is to see to it that our guests come to understand and respect their bodies' strengths and limitations and to learn to heal and strengthen their bodies in order to enjoy maximum physiological health.

The guests who enroll in the Life Enhancement Program are a pretty sophisticated group. These people know that exercise is crucial to health, and they know that, if their bodies are not functioning well or if they are experiencing pain, something needs to change. They come to Canyon Ranch ready to dig into the whys and hows of movement. They want to find out how they develop the skills, abilities, and daily habits to minimize—and even reverse—many of the physical limitations and ailments we commonly associate with aging. They come for the astonishingly beautiful natural environment of Canyon Ranch, and they arrive with a willingness to participate in many types of fitness programs and classes. But along with that, they also learn a lot about how their bodies—and particularly their joints and muscles—work.

When guests leave Canyon Ranch, they have renewed respect for their bodies. They're excited by what they've discovered about their bodies—especially how wonderful they can feel with healthy living. They leave our program ready to really *move* into life.

The purpose of this book is to bring that experience to you.

INTRODUCTION

When was the last time you went out to play? A lot of people find this question to be a little ridiculous, but I do think it is worth pondering. When we're kids, we run, jump, climb, and scramble effortlessly and joyously—and pretty much all the time. Who among us doesn't remember how alive we felt when we slid into home plate, landed our first cartwheel, or ran all-out until we fell into the grass, gasping for air?

When we're children, our bodies are *primed* to move—every ligament, tendon, and muscle is supple and receptive. Then we age, and our desire to move like this may diminish. But our body's ability doesn't necessarily have to! We health professionals who specialize in movement and fitness are learning that it's not our bodies that compel us to slow down or stop enjoying what we used to do. Rather, it's our conscious connection to our bodies that diminishes. And that's a big part of what makes us "feel old"—when we don't have to at all!

The implications of this fact are profound: It is common wisdom that movement is medicine. Everyone knows that exercise is crucial to supporting good health. What most of us don't know, however, is that movement is also the key to minimizing—or even eliminating—many of the physical ailments associated with aging. I happen to know, firsthand, that a 59-year-old man can live an active, joyful, and challenging lifestyle. Because that's who I am. And that's the lifestyle I lead.

But I also know that this feeling about life, and this joy in motion and activity, is not the exclusive domain of a physical therapist at Canyon Ranch. The hundreds of visitors who have come and gone have discovered that this is within *their* reach, too. And I know that there are millions more—most likely including you, the reader of this book—who can also feel this way about their body, their lifestyle, and their outlook on the years ahead.

Among the many guests who come to the Life Enhancement Program, there are quite a number of former athletes who miss the part of their lives when they were keenly engaged in their favorite sports. While recognizing that they will not set the personal records that they attained before, they want to bring sports back into their lives wisely and reasonably.

Others come to us having battled debilitating diseases, such as heart disease, diabetes, or cancer. They are committed to living the rest of their lives at optimal health, and they know that physical wellness and performance are key to this.

And there are still others who come to us simply because they know something is missing (that word *play* comes to mind again) and they can't quite identify what it is. So, yes, our guests run the gamut of fitness levels and ages, yet they all have one thing in common: a willingness to think differently about how their bodies work and what their bodies just might actually be capable of.

POETRY IN MOTION

I've been a physical therapist for 13 years and worked in fitness for 32, and I'm still in awe when I see how beautiful the human body is when it's in motion. When I see a child skipping, an older man walking with dignity and ease, or a young mother balancing a child on one hip and a bag of groceries on the other, I marvel at how strong, supple, and versatile our bodies are. Think about it: We are, in essence, nothing more than bone, fluid, and muscle (with a few organs thrown in). How is it that our bodies can do so many things? It is a question that I continue to enjoy exploring.

But our bodies certainly aren't invincible. Many of us live with some sort of pain or discomfort. Some just feel it from time to time; others have chronic pain that they wake up to every morning and take to bed with them at night. (Pain, in fact—of all kinds—is what motivates many people to come to Canyon Ranch in the first place.)

A good number of people who experience almost nonstop discomfort seem to have the belief that this is "just the way it is." I help them discover otherwise—in the same way that I hope I can help you begin to find a pain-free lifestyle if that's what's troubling you. Our joints and muscles (which hang elegantly on our skeletons) are fragile in some ways, but they are also highly resilient and receptive to repair. Though serious injuries may need intensive medical intervention, many times people experience substantial healing and recovery if they just have a willingness to think about movement differently.

And *move* is what our bodies are meant to do.

CAN YOU PUT YOURSELF ON "HOLD"?

If you think it's easy to stay motionless, you should try it sometime. I mean really try it.

Here's an experiment. Turn off your television, radio, and computer. Sit down with a clock or watch within view. Once you've read these instructions, put this book down. Then . . .

Do not move a muscle for 5 full minutes. I mean a muscle. Do not blink, scratch, twitch, or touch anything. Think you can do it?

I bet not. Our bodies (even when we are asleep) are in constant motion. Not only that, but when they are still, they *want* to move. So if you start moving, you're not "restless" or "nervous" or "stir-crazy" or anything like that. You're just going along with what your body wants to do!

When I was new to the field of physical therapy, I worked part-time in a nursing home. We visited and worked with very elderly patients, many of whom were confined to beds and wheelchairs. Some shuffled along behind walkers. Very few could easily get to their feet and walk around freely.

And I wondered: Where were the *mobile* elderly people? And was the immobility of all these people an inevitable fact of aging?

In 1990, William J. Evans addressed this very question. Evans had worked with a population of nursing home adults with an average age of 90 years. He put them on a high-intensity, strength-training program for 60 days. The results were nothing short of miraculous: At the end of those 2 months, the strength of the residents improved, on average, 174 percent. Muscle mass and mobility increased along with strength. The conclusion? Slowing down and losing our muscle mass and our mobility are *not* the result of aging: They are due to a lack of use.

In other studies, researchers working with middle-aged men and women have found that people who have just 10 days of bed rest show a sharp decrease in aerobic capacity. In fact, in the groups studied, 10 days of relative immobility turned out to be the equivalent of 5 to 10 years of aging. This kind of dramatic example shows us, unequivocally, the toll a lack of activity and movement can take on a person—regardless of chronological age.

MUSCLES: NOT JUST FOR THE MACHO

Muscle is, quite literally, worth its weight in gold. Our muscles, when they are strong, well nourished, and used regularly, are what power us through life. They lift us and propel us forward. Muscles are what allow us to be more than just an inert bag of bones and water that wobbles across the floor.

It's been estimated that the average American adult loses ½ pound of muscle each year. This isn't because our bodies are designed to shed this tissue—it's because we don't move enough to maintain our muscle mass. (If you've ever broken a bone, you know how weak and atrophied the limb around a fracture looks after the cast is removed; this is due to disuse of the muscles in that limb! You also know that resuming the routine tasks of daily life will begin to plump up those frozen muscles again.)

The great thing about muscle (which is living, breathing tissue) is that it is highly regenerative. Muscles need to be used and to be used on a regular basis. That's why movement and muscle go hand in hand.

ACTIVITY VERSUS EXERCISE

I'd like to take a moment to discuss what may seem obvious, but what has a profound impact on our understanding of movement and health. We all know that the Centers for Disease Control and Prevention (commonly referred to as the CDC) recommends that we engage in at least (or strive to engage in) 30 minutes of moderate activity a day, or 20 minutes of vigorous activity three times a week.

What does this mean?

Many of us groan when we're reminded of this recommendation, believing we are meant to hit the gym every day—and that we somehow fail if we don't. This isn't at all what the CDC is advocating. Nor do I. Every time you purposefully move your body, you are being active. Your type of movement may be defined as "moderate" or "vigorous"—I'll help you decide which—but no matter what, it's still activity.

In other words, don't underestimate the physical benefits you get when you lug a 10-pound basket of laundry down to your basement, wash it, fold it, and lug it back upstairs. When you engage in a task like this, you're active! And your body will thank you.

A Sampling of Moderate-Intensity Activity

INDOORS	OUTDOORS	INDOORS OR OUTDOORS
• Dancing, general (Greek, hula, flamenco, Middle Eastern and swing) • Riding a stationary bike • Actively playing with children • Taking Jazzercise • Scrubbing the floor	• Mowing lawn, general • Frisbee playing, general • Playing golf, walking the course • Shoveling light snow • Downhill skiing with light effort • Raking leaves • Hand washing/waxing a car	• Playing basketball, shooting hoops • Walking, brisk pace (mall/around a track/treadmill) • Doing water aerobics • Jogging/walking combination (In a 30-minute period, you should be jogging for fewer than 10 minutes.)

Published by the CDC, Centers for Disease Control and Prevention, a division of the Department of Health and Human Services

I always find it helpful to remind my clients that they can break down the daily 30-minute goal into smaller, easier chunks of time and it will be just as beneficial. Walking briskly to and from work for 15 minutes each way counts, as does riding a stationary bike for 10 minutes, three times a day. The point is to strive for *conscious* activity for a half hour every day. If you do this, the benefits will be immeasurable.

Some adults do love going to the gym. Parents, especially, may have discovered that this is a chance to enjoy some much-needed quiet time and to reconnect with oneself, while also toning and strengthening up. Or the attraction might be the chance to engage in a group activity, such as a dance or yoga class. But moving inside a gym is no better—from a physiological standpoint—than hiking up a lovely slope, taking a dip in that summer pond, or playing a quick game of tag with your grandkids in the front yard.

Activity *is* exercise—it's just spontaneous, unstructured, and informal.

For many of us, especially as we age, adopting a more formal form of activity—engaging in an exercise plan—can be quite beneficial, and at times, it can be literally life-saving. And I know, because I've devoted my life to designing programs specifically for people who haven't been able to be as physically active as they'd like.

One of the goals of this book (and of my life's work) is to show people that activity and exercise go hand in hand. One is not necessarily more beneficial than the other. Ideally, we'd all engage in both forms of movement, knowing that everyday activity, coupled with appropriate types of structured exercise, will bring us to optimal health and keep us in our prime for life!

ACKNOWLEDGMENTS

Prime for Life originated in the mind of Meredith Blevins, who recruited my help for a book on fitness for baby boomers. It would not have been possible without her. I will be forever grateful to Meredith and her husband, Win Blevins, for their support and friendship and gift of this opportunity. Meredith was responsible for much of the writing, laughter, and spiritual guidance. She was my partner in crime for most of the project. I may owe my current sanity to Meredith and Win for their support during the tough times in writing this book.

Emily Heckman made some changes to the manuscript. Edward B. Claflin provided wonderful, insightful editing help in the final stages. He helped me rediscover the original voice that Meredith started.

This book would not have been possible without the extraordinary faculty of the physical therapy department of Washington University in St. Louis. Many ideas in this book are due to their genius. Movement Impairment Diagnoses, touched on lightly in *Prime for Life*, were conceived by Shirley A. Sahrmann, PT, PhD. Her insights in showing each patient how faulty movement patterns provide potentially more powerful diagnoses than traditional medical ones has dramatically improved physical therapy care. Barbara J. Norton, PT, PhD, deserves thanks for patience in my academic work. Special thanks, too, go to Michael J. Mueller, PT, PhD, for extraordinary patience in awaiting a long overdue paper and for inspiring a key concept in *Prime for Life*. His Physical Stress Theory powerfully shows that individuals have a significant choice regarding maintaining health of all tissues.

To Mel and Enid Zuckerman, founders of Canyon Ranch Health Resort, I owe 27 years of thanks. They provided me with the best job I could have ever envisioned. In this magical place, I get to work with amazing health-care providers and meet wonderful people who come from all over the world. Every day in the Life Enhancement Center is an adventure of brave people striving to be open to the possibility of change.

Finally, I will be eternally grateful to my beloved family, Lynne and Tyler for giving me time to write this book.

PRIME FOR LIFE

CHAPTER ONE

MOVEMENT AS MEDICINE

"Lack of activity destroys the good
condition of every human being, while
movement and methodical physical
exercise save it and preserve it."

—*Plato*

I think it's generally understood that exercise is crucial for maintaining good health. But it's worth pointing out some of the "extra" physiological benefits of staying active that move beyond muscle strength and joint and tendon health. Let's have a look.

Right now, if you were to get up out of your seat and walk into the next room and back, a whole host of processes would be activated throughout your body that would bring you countless health benefits. With just a few steps, you would initiate subtle changes in your breathing, your heart rate, your adrenal system, and your brain, to name a few—on top of the changes and benefits you'd be getting by activating your musculoskeletal system. You'd also be likely to lower your stress level and prompt your body to release hormones that will strengthen your immune system and boost your overall health and sense of well-being.

Being physically active on a regular basis:

- ○ Promotes heart health
- ○ Sharpens (and protects) your brain
- ○ Reduces stress
- ○ Is key to losing weight
- ○ Will improve your sex life
- ○ Protects against—and reverses the damage of—diabetes

MOVING FOR A HEALTHIER HEART

Let's start with the benefits to the heart.

The heart is a muscle. And, like all muscles, it thrives when it is really put to work regularly. Few people know it, but inactivity is actually one of the leading causes of coronary artery disease, the name for any heart-related problem—ranging from angina and arrhythmia to fatal heart attacks—which is caused by problems with the arteries leading from the heart. Early in life, the risks of inactivity begin to build steadily. (For instance, a recent report warns that children need at least 90 minutes a day of physical activity if they want to avoid being in the high-risk group for heart disease when they become adults.)

People who exercise regularly and at high intensity have the lowest risk of developing heart disease. Indeed, a person who maintains an active lifestyle has a 45 percent lower risk of developing heart disease than a sedentary person.

When we are exerting ourselves physically, we pump oxygen into our hearts, which expands the blood vessels and arteries, allowing blood to flow efficiently and freely through them. Exercise also improves cholesterol and lipid levels, further protecting us from heart disease. Regular exercise also stimulates the immune system to decrease proteins that help cause plaque buildup in the arteries and to increase the proteins that prevent it.

When people come into the Life Enhancement Program at Canyon Ranch, they often have a ton of questions about heart health. We ask all Canyon Ranch guests to check in with a nurse to assess their readiness for exercise. Often they are encouraged to see one of our physicians for a cardiac stress test to determine their optimum level of exertion.

The fitness staff and I are all experts at teaching pacing for optimum benefit and enjoyment. Here's an example:

One morning I took a group of new guests out for a walk. My group consisted of three men and three women, with an age range between 35 and 70. I told them that we were going to walk a 4-mile loop that would incorporate some hills, most of which were gentle slopes, but a couple of which were pretty steep.

I like to talk to my guests as I'm walking, not only to be efficient with our time, but also to show them that being able to walk and talk is a good thing. When you can carry on a comfortable conversation while walking for any significant duration, it means that you're not overexerting yourself. (Exercising more rigorously is also beneficial, but when I'm working with a group that's just beginning to look at walking in a new way, I always advocate for moderation at first.)

Before the walk, we discussed pacing and the overall health benefits of walking. Again, as we struck off, I reminded everyone that this wasn't a race—that all members would, after the first mile, gradually work their way up to their own, comfortable walking speed.

Almost immediately, a very fit woman named Sarah, who was in her late sixties, established herself as the leader of our group. She walked at a brisk pace and obviously enjoyed it—her relaxed smile and bright eyes told the story. Because she kept getting ahead of us, going at her own pace, I had her loop back periodically to keep the group together.

Sarah had an easy gait. As she walked, I could see her body was nicely aligned and relaxed. Letting her continue at her established pace, I stayed back with the rest of the group to coach them.

At the back of the pack was a man in his late thirties named Jim, who was moderately obese and clearly out of shape. As I watched Jim struggle along, I noticed that he kept looking at Sarah as she got ahead of us, then circled back, rejoined us, and went ahead. Something about her pace seemed to be a direct threat to him.

Once we reached the 1-mile mark, I encouraged everyone to find their groove and to walk along at their own pace.

Then we came to the first rather steep hill. Sarah, never breaking her stride, began to walk up the hill. At that point, Jim, who had begun sweating profusely and was dabbing his forehead with a bandana, picked up his pace to follow her. I ran a bit to catch up with him.

"Are you okay, Jim?" I asked.

He was clearly laboring hard. "It's been a while," he panted, "I just need to find my stride."

I asked Jim if he wouldn't mind stopping at the top of the hill, and he breathlessly gave me the "okay" sign. I then waited while the other walkers all made their way up the same slope. Once I got to the top, I was alone with Jim (everyone else had continued to walk on). I stood beside him and offered him a drink of water.

"Why are you trying so hard?" I asked him.

At first, his response was a bit defensive: "I'm not trying hard! I'm just getting warmed up."

I waited a moment (and gave him a chance to catch his breath and for his heart rate to go down some). Then I said, "Jim, I'm going to make you have a good time if it's the last thing I do—*not* the last thing *you* do."

He looked at me with surprise, and then laughed.

I proceeded to continue, "We're here to move and to feel good—not to run ourselves ragged."

He smiled and nodded. After resting for a few more minutes, we walked the remaining 3 miles, engaged in one of the most delightful conversations I'd had in some time.

The next morning, Jim arrived for another walk and this time, he smiled and waved to me from the back of the pack. It is joy that brings you back to exercise—not pain or suffering.

A FIT BODY DOES A BRAIN GOOD

The brain is a remarkable organ, not just because of its vast potential and sophistication, but because, like muscle, it can be strengthened and repaired throughout our lifetime. And this is exciting news for all of us who plan on staying in our prime for decades to come.

I love sharing this tidbit of our evolution with my clients: Did you know that our brains (which are part of our nervous system) evolved specifically to *coordinate movement*? Our primitive bodies needed a central processing center, where nerves would receive and transmit information so that we could move around in the world. The primitive brains of all living creatures—including humans—were designed so that we would be able to react (flee from danger) or act (hunt and gather). That way, we were active, having an impact on the world around us, rather than sitting around waiting to see what would happen next. (No one wants to be someone else's lunch!) So remember: Our brains have evolved specifically to work in concert with our nerves and muscles in order to keep us in motion.

Until very recent years it was thought that the adult brain, once formed, did not significantly change throughout the years—except for the kind of gradual decline in memory power that we eventually experience. Now we know better. At any stage of life, our brains continue to change and respond to new learning. Exercise improves that process. Not only that, but exercise also helps prevent age-related cognitive decline—better known as memory loss—in a number of powerful ways.

In one study, 27 people were subjected to three kinds of "activities"—(1) high-impact running sprints, (2) low-impact aerobics, or (3) a period of rest. Immediately after each of the activities, they were given the task of learning unfamiliar vocabulary words. Their ability to remember the words was tested 1 week later and again more than 8 months later.

Researchers reported that the participants' speed of vocabulary learning was 20 percent higher after running (activity #1) than it was after low-impact aerobics (#2) or rest (#3). Remembrance of the words was also significantly better in the first group. In addition, the runners had higher levels of brain-derived neurotropin factor, a key brain chemical associated with brain development. They also had higher neurotransmitter levels, which correlated to improved learning.

Similar findings came from the Nurses' Health Study, which tracked exercise habits and cognitive function in more than 18,000 women aged 70 to 81. The fittest, most active women had a 20 percent lower risk for cognitive decline than sedentary women. One and a half hours of easy walking per day significantly correlated to better mental function and less decline with age.

A HABIT OF EXERCISE

Did you know that the word *exercise* actually derives in part from a Latin word that means "to maintain, to keep, to ward off"? The etymology of this word ties in perfectly with the effect exercise has on our brains. Movement and activity truly do "ward off" the ill effects of aging.

Several studies show that simply walking is a great way to invigorate your brain. Because walking isn't overly strenuous, all the blood and oxygen that are circulating through your body are available to your brain (rather than going to, say, the muscles in legs that might be pounding the pavement). Maybe that's why we're told to "walk it off" when we're upset or we take a walk when we want to clear our heads.

Walking regularly improves memory and also wards off stroke. In improving cholesterols and fat profiles in the blood, exercise decreases blockage in the brain as it does in the heart. When you are challenging your brain with new movement patterns in that dance class or new sport, you are optimizing brain function too.

Bottom line? Anytime you engage in physical activity, your brain is getting a boost. So remember, if you want to keep remembering, keep moving!

EXERCISE SOOTHES YOUR SOUL

Many people believe that when they're stressed out, the best remedy is to hole up and become inactive. This couldn't be further from the truth. Engaging in a brisk walk or an exercise class will not only tone your body, but it will also protect your body (and mind) from the ravages of stress.

Stress, in its most elemental form, is a normal physiological response to danger. Our body releases the hormones we need to react appropriately (this is called the "fight-or-flight" response). Naturally, we need to fight or flee if we're about to be attacked. But when stress is chronic—when we feel like fighting or fleeing nearly all the time—something not quite right is going on. Our bodies are being flooded with hormones such as cortisol. Although it helps prepare us for the struggle or flight from danger by increasing blood sugar levels, it also depresses the immune system, making us more prone to illness and less able to heal from injuries. In someone who is already predisposed to developing diabetes, chronically high blood sugar levels fuel the problem.

When stress is chronic, all sorts of physical damage can occur. Our cells may weaken. Blood pressure becomes elevated. The immune system loses some of its ability to fight off bacteria and viruses.

Exercise combats the damage caused by stress. When we exercise, our bodies release counterbalancing soothing hormones (endorphins and the like) into our bloodstream. These calming hormones are responsible for that legendary runner's high, a yogi's sense of serenity, and a tennis player's moving into the zone.

Being physically fit calms our nerves, allows us to get a better night's sleep, and keeps our brains sharp and ready for anything. There is, quite simply, no better stress buster. Being fitter means literally that it takes more stress—either the physical or emotional kind—to trigger the stress response.

MOVING THE POUNDS OFF

We all know that dietary calorie restriction and exercise go hand in hand—but why? It's not that exercising guarantees you greater weight loss (it won't); it's because if you reduce your caloric intake *without* exercise, your body sheds both fat and muscle, which is not a good thing. When we lose muscle, our metabolism slows down considerably (that's another way of saying our bodies go into starvation mode). And it becomes even harder to lose weight (not to mention do pretty much anything else).

Engaging in physical activity of any kind will help you get leaner and stay that way. Any cardiovascular exercise will burn calories, which is the key to weight loss. It doesn't matter whether you swim, bike, walk, or run. As long as you expend more energy than you consume, you will get leaner. The key is finding some kind of movement that brings you pleasure. Once you discover that, it's almost a guarantee that you'll do that movement regularly.

Exercising rigorously also elevates your metabolism and encourages your body to burn calories more efficiently, which means it burns more, faster. And this, too, helps you lose excess fat.

You have likely heard the adage that muscle weighs more than fat. Although this just *can't* be true (a pound, after all, is a pound), muscle is more dense and compact than fat, and so it takes up much less space in your body. That's why, if you build muscle, you may not lose any pounds, but you will lose inches, and your clothes may become looser. And, lo and behold, you will look as though you have lost weight, because you have denser muscle tissue!

PACING YOURSELF—
OPTIMAL EXERCISE INTENSITY

Some experts use the "predicted maximum heart rate" to help people estimate how hard they should work when they're engaging in cardiovascular exercise (that is, the kind of exercise that gets your heart pumping well above resting rate).

The calculation is a mathematical relationship, based on age. Just subtract your age from 220 to get the predicted maximum heart rate. Using this method, a 40-year-old would have a "maximum" heart rate of 220 minus 40, which equals 180 beats per minute. Then, if you want to find out the "moderate" exercise heart rate—where you want to be most of the time—multiply this by 70 percent (or 0.70). So for a 40-year-old, the "moderate" exercise heart rate is about 126 beats per minute.

Here's how this helps you pace yourself. If, after a slow, progressive 5- to 10-

minute warmup, your heart rate is below 126 beats per minute, you would speed up or (if you're on a treadmill, for instance) climb a steeper grade. If you're well over 126 beats per minute, you know your heart rate needs to slow down (and so does your pace or level of incline) if you're going to be maintaining a moderate pace.

Heart rate is the most accurate way to determine optimal exercise intensity. But the predicted values are, unfortunately, based on averages among Americans. Individually, our "maximum" and "moderate" heart rates can vary significantly from these predicted values. (Many blood pressure and heart medications can also make a difference in how you want to pace yourself.) So, even though you can use predicted maximum heart rate calculations as a ballpark estimate, there are still advantages to having a cardiac stress test.

For one thing, a stress test is always done in the presence of a doctor who is qualified to interpret the test. In the end, you'll not only find out your maximum and moderate heart rate levels, but you'll also walk away with an assessment of your heart health and fitness level.

ANOTHER MEASUREMENT TO GO BY

The Borg Perceived Exertion Scale (BPES) is another way to help you find out how to pace yourself. It is about 90 percent accurate in determining someone's level of exercise intensity.

The BPES uses a numeric scale of 6 to 20. Level 6 is sitting in a chair, relaxed. Level 20 is maximal exertion, not sustainable. (This is equivalent to being 10 years old and racing your best friend as hard as you can across a big field—competing to the point of collapse.) Most people will describe 11 as "light" intensity. This would correspond to 60 percent of your actual maximum heart rate. To get an idea of this pace or intensity, you can use the "conversation" test I mentioned before. If you can exercise while you easily carry on a conversation using big words and long sentences without being noticeably out of breath, you're at level 11.

At level 13 on the Borg scale, most people will describe their intensity as "pleasantly moderate." They will be able to converse in short sentences and be just a tad out of breath. They will sound slightly "huffy-puffy."

At level 15, you'll feel like the exercise is "heavy" or "very hard." Most people will only be able to speak in short phrases and will sound very winded.

Using the Borg scale, then, you can determine your "moderate" level fairly easily. It's likely that this level is very close to what a doctor or physical therapist would call "moderate" after giving you a stress test. And it might be very close to the calculation of "moderate" that you arrive at doing the math for your predicted maximum heart rate.

What it amounts to is this: moderate, for most people, is a comfortable and

MODIFIED BORG
PERCEIVED EXERTION SCALE

6	Sitting in a chair, relaxed ....
7	Very, very light intensity ....
8	....
9	Very light intensity...
10	....
11	Light intensity (easy to converse in long sentences) ....
12	....
13	Somewhat hard, "Moderate" intensity (can speak in short breathy sentences)
14	....
15	Hard, "Heavy" intensity (can speak very breathy phrases or a few words)
16	....
17	Very hard intensity ....
18	....
19	....
20	All out! Not sustainable...

effective intensity of exercise. It almost doesn't feel like exercise. That's where you want to be.

If that seems counterintuitive—if you're asking yourself, "How can I really get anywhere if I just do moderate exercise?"—just consider this. Which do you think is better for weight loss or getting fit: a periodic killer workout that burns tons of calories, but which you dread repeating, or a pleasantly invigorating one during which you can enjoy conversation and take pleasure in your surroundings?

Occasional vigorous workouts for healthy people can optimize their fitness. That said, most days, I recommend "moderate." (For individuals with high blood pressure, the consensus is that light to moderate works best.) For instance, the kinds of walks that are done at a moderate pace—at *your own moderate* pace—are what I call "pleasure walks." They are enjoyable and almost spiritual in that they connect you to the world and encourage contemplation and conversation.

BEING ACTIVE IS SEXY

When we think of our sexual ideal, most of us think of someone who is successful, physically fit, and clearly in his or her prime. Being sexy isn't necessarily about looking younger or being a cougar out on the market; it's about feeling great and being comfortable and content in your own skin. It's about being excited by physicality and health. Sex is a pretty rigorous activity!

Human beings are wired for intimate contact, and nothing makes that more satisfying than having a body that is strong, supple, and healthy.

MOVING AWAY FROM DIABETES (A MOVE WE ALL NEED TO MAKE)

Clearly, exercising regularly can help prevent or combat a whole host of illnesses, but given that obesity, being sedentary, and getting diabetes all go hand in hand (and are at record levels—we're truly experiencing an epidemic of all three), diabetes is worth a special mention here.

Diabetes is the condition in which our bodies lose their ability to process sugar (glucose) and become, in essence, poisoned by sugar. Too much sugar in our bloodstreams breaks down cells, wears out nerves, throws our entire endocrine (hormone) system out of whack, and generally wreaks havoc on our bodies. People who suffer from diabetes and don't treat it aggressively run the

THE VIAGRA OF EXERCISE

Here it is—hard evidence that plenty of exercise (plus a few other factors) can improve men's sex lives.

In a study conducted in Italy, researchers selected a number of men who had problems with erectile dysfunction (ED)—in layman's terms, failure to get an erection when an erection was called for. (Significantly, all the men were overweight; obesity is a risk factor for ED.) The men were divided into two groups. Half received information about healthy living, but without any other follow-through. The other half went on a 2-year, proactive lifestyle program that was similar to what we recommend at Canyon Ranch. These men were asked to do an hour of cardiovascular exercise each day and worked with an exercise trainer once a month. (At the same time, they were placed on a healthy eating program and they checked in monthly with a dietician.)

The participants were tested and measured for fitness at the beginning and end of the study. After 2 years, the active group reported a 31 percent improvement in sexual function. All the evidence pointed to a direct correlation between fitness and normal sexual function.

Their blood tests, which were regularly monitored in the study, provide one important clue to these happy results. Testing showed signs of improved nitric oxide function in their vessels. Nitric oxide just happens to be a chemical—found naturally inside our bodies—that causes the dilation of veins and arteries, obviously important in getting an erection. The miracle medications—Viagra, Cialis, and Levitra—provide help to men with erectile dysfunction (ED) by improving their sensitivity to nitric oxide.

Sure, exercise might not be as fast acting as these renowned medications, but this study is just further proof that small changes can make a big difference in your life—including your love life.

risk of developing a wide array of secondary conditions, including heart disease, nerve damage, vision loss (even blindness), vascular disease, kidney failure, and stroke.

What are the most effective treatments for diabetes? Changing your diet and engaging in regular, significant (meaning moderate to vigorous intensity) exercise.

A change in diet might seem obvious because we all know certain foods have an impact on blood sugar levels. But how does exercise combat diabetes?

Here's what happens. When we exercise, we help our muscles extract glucose (blood sugar) from our bloodstream (where it's been stuck). We also help our bodies do a better job of metabolizing insulin, which is the hormone responsible for transporting glucose from our bloodstream into our cells, where it can be used as fuel.

Here are some incredibly motivating facts about exercise and diabetes that ought to be of interest to all of us who want to control it—or prevent its onset:

○ One workout improves the body's sensitivity to insulin for up to 36 hours. (You get optimum blood sugar control if you are active— in the ways I'm advocating—five or six days per week.)

○ Our risk of getting diabetes increases each year after the age of 35. But research has shown that men in their sixties who are master endurance athletes have the same insulin and glucose profiles as young, elite athletes. This suggests that the risk of diabetes isn't related as closely to age as it is to activity level.

○ Diabetes is often considered to be a disease of "overweight" people. But the research on master athletes found inactive men had higher insulin levels at all ages—and that included inactive men who were lean rather than overweight. Older, leaner men also had elevated glucose levels.

○ During exercise, a person with diabetes often experiences a dramatic drop in glucose levels. This indicates that exercise is helping move the glucose from the blood into the cells and muscles, where it belongs (their fuel is glucose!). During exercise, your muscle cells use glucose without needing insulin.

Samantha's
STORY

Afew years ago, a woman named Samantha came for an extended stay at the Life Enhancement Program. Sam, as she asked us to call her, weighed 250 pounds and had recently been diagnosed with diabetes. With a loving husband, terrific kids, and a successful business at home, she had come to Canyon Ranch for some serious self-reckoning.

"Getting the diabetes diagnosis was the wake-up I've needed," she confided. "I knew I couldn't go on like this."

Samantha opted for a full workup with our medical director. A stress test revealed no cardiac problems. She also checked in with our dieticians. She said she wanted to work to get back to her "fighting weight," which had been 145 pounds when she got married.

Finally, she came to me. I put Sam on a standard, reasonable starting program, where she'd walk on a treadmill for 25 minutes. Together, we set a goal for her, which was that we would gradually increase the incline on the treadmill to a grade of 10 to 15 percent without her becoming winded. She was skeptical, telling me she hated hills. "Do you live in a hilly area?" I asked. She acknowledged that she did, but I told her that the incline wasn't the problem or the risk. It was inappropriate pacing—not the hill, but the speed on elevation that caused her to overwork. Every week in the program I teach people this simple pacing technique that makes hills safe and fun. I told her that with each rise in elevation, if she became short of breath, she should slow the speed more.

Before Sam started, I put a heart rate monitor on her. I set the monitor to send an alert signal if Sam's heart rate exceeded 70 percent of the maximum established by her stress test.

Sam began to walk. And, shortly, to huff and puff. Then the heart rate monitor went off. I urged her to slow down and she did—for about 30 seconds. Then the monitor went off again.

We went back and forth like that—Beep! "Slow down." Beep! "Slow down!" Beep!—until I was able to convince her to truly maintain the slowed-down pace.

"But I'm only going 1.1 miles per hour!" she groaned.

"Who are you trying to beat?" I replied.

In time, as the treadmill's incline began to rise, Sam realized that pacing herself and taking it slow wasn't such a bad thing. She was able to stay with it, even up a steep incline. By the time she got to 15 percent, a very steep hill, she was only going 0.7 miles per hour, but she was feeling good and was very encouraged that she could walk anywhere and like it.

Afterward, she stepped off the treadmill, smiled at me, and said, "I really enjoyed that! I thought I hated walking up hills."

I heard this every day for the next month. When Sam left Canyon Ranch, she had increased her walk to an hour and was 8 pounds lighter. Her glucose levels were much more stable, and she had a fitness and lifestyle plan in hand. Most important, she had learned that a pleasant, moderate pace made exercise enjoyable. And it was a finding that she could take back home. Sam lived in a hilly area, but she had usually avoided the hills. With her experience at Canyon Ranch, she learned that walking need not be limited to flat terrain to be enjoyable. Whatever the steepness of a hill, she discovered how she could walk at a moderate pace that was just right for her.

That is the key to long-term, regular activity.

Six months after Sam paid her first visit to Canyon Ranch, she came back for a 1-week "tune-up." When I saw her again, she looked radiant—and 20 pounds lighter! Clearly, she was following her take-home plan well.

When Sam shared her new medical records with me, I was thrilled to see that her glucose and insulin levels had improved significantly.

She was still taking some medications—as she had previously—but I saw that the doses had been reduced. I loved seeing her progress.

Samantha continued to come back to Canyon Ranch regularly. By the third year, she was a woman transformed. She had reached her goal weight of 145 pounds. She looked so much younger than her 57 years! And she was off all medication for her diabetes. Even though she no longer came to the Life Enhancement center regularly (she checked into the main resort), we'd see each other while out hiking or playing a game of tennis. We always hugged warmly, reveling in our shared commitment to being fit and healthy.

GET THE PACE RIGHT

The secret of being a successful walker—one who enjoys walking fast on flat terrain and up any hill—is appropriate pacing.

Always warm up by gradually increasing speed for 5 to 10 minutes. On level terrain, train to increase speed by doing three to six 1-minute intervals walking as fast as you can, swinging your arms and focusing on smooth, quiet heel-to-toe rolling of the feet. (If you're noisily slapping down your feet as you walk, it means you're not making adequate use of your shin muscles.)

In between speedy, 1-minute intervals, slow down to allow the muscles to recover.

When you ascend any hill, pacing is crucial. On a treadmill, for example, decrease the speed by about 0.2 miles per hour for each 1 percent increase in the grade. Outside, just focus on your breathing. If you can't carry on a conversation in short sentences without being very out of breath, slow down. On a very steep hill, if you're just starting out, this might mean pausing on each step to take a few breaths. If you do that, you will be walking much slower, but continuing to experience that feeling of pleasant invigoration that, over time, leads to faster speeds, higher fitness levels, and a significantly leaner body.

MOVING IMPROVES YOUR MOOD

This is the last major point I'm going to make about the benefits of being fit and active, before really diving into the nitty-gritty of what this book is all about—getting fit and feeling fabulous by understanding how your muscles, joints, and ligaments work.

At this point, it really is worth reminding all of you readers that the biggest benefit you'll get from being active is a sense of well-being.

Those of us who are committed to maintaining—and building on—our level of physical fitness gain so much emotional benefit from it that it's almost hard to put it into words. But let me try.

Being physically fit:

○ Makes you feel up to the challenges of life, whether you're walking to work when the subway is late and knowing you'll still be on time, or entering and finishing your first triathlon. No mountain seems too steep, no valley too deep when you feel strong, healthy, and fit.

○ Is "my beauty secret" (as one of my female clients put it). Have you ever noticed how much better you feel and look in your clothes when you're in good shape? How much straighter you stand? How much clearer your skin is (not to mention your thoughts are)? Feeling healthy and fit—and reaping the physical rewards of it—will definitely elevate your outlook.

○ Can help you sleep better at night. And that's critically important! Sleep is crucial to overall good health and maintaining a high-functioning immune system. Studies show that postmenopausal women who work out for 30 minutes each morning (the time of day is important) sleep much more restfully than those who are sedentary. (Exercising vigorously late in the day or near bedtime is not, however, conducive to a better night's sleep for anyone. After exercising, most people need at least 3 or 4 hours to wind down.)

○ Will improve your sex life. (Wait. Have I already said this? Very well, this one is always worth repeating.)

It has been said that cardiovascular exercise is more powerful than any single antidepressant for the alleviation of mild to moderate depression. In one study, 156 people with major depression were randomly separated into three groups— (1) those who received an antidepressant medication, (2) those who went on a regular aerobic exercise routine, and (3) a group that did both, exercised regularly and received the antidepressant.

When the outcome of the study was analyzed, researchers learned that the people on the antidepressant improved faster at first. But after 16 weeks, researchers concluded, there was no difference in outcomes among the three groups.

Regular aerobic exercise, by itself, was just as effective in treating mild to moderate depression as taking an antidepressant.

Exercise is one powerful tool to bring joy into your life. Cardiovascular exercise has been found to increase production of serotonin, norepinephrine, and dopamine, brain chemicals that the leading antidepressants affect. In the end, no one disputes the benefit of exercise for overall physical as well as mental health. And I often find that clients who spent their thirties and forties cooped up at a desk or not prioritizing their health and bodies feel better and younger in their fifties and beyond when they adopt the activities, exercise, and movement that promote their bodies' prime.

When you exercise regularly and safely, you'll likely find yourself feeling prime for life, too.

CHAPTER TWO

GETTING STARTED

*"Every body perseveres in its state of being
at rest or of moving uniformly straight
forward, except insofar as it is compelled
to change its state by force impressed."*

—*Newton's Law of Inertia*

We've all heard the expression "a body in motion stays in motion" and can thank the immortal physicist Sir Isaac Newton for pointing this out to us. I hope you'll subscribe to this law. It's actually very easy. Once you get in motion, you'll stay in motion.

Still, the physical activity I'm about to describe may be new to you. And with anything new, getting started is *always* the hardest part. Many of us are simply put off or even become tired when we think of exercise. A lot of us were injured somewhere along the way and our confidence in our bodies has been diminished. Still others of us simply feel that getting fit requires some sort of expertise that we just don't have, and we're at a loss as to how to get it.

It's human nature, I think, to put up internal roadblocks before we start something new. But here's the great thing about being more active: You can mull over all your doubts, misgivings, and questions about it while you're in motion! It really is that simple.

There are a few basic things we all must take into consideration before beginning any new activity. First of all, you need to decide "where you are" and what your *personal* goal is in this prime for life program. For some, this may be an activity such as reclaiming the ability to walk up several flights of stairs without pain or without becoming breathless. For others, this may mean beginning the rigorous endurance training needed to take on a dangerous, high-altitude mountain climb.

I'm going to take a few minutes and outline what some of those issues may be. Having a sense of "where you are" in terms of your own unique ability is key to upping your activity level in ways that will not only offer you the highest reward, but will also *stick*, so that you truly do become a body in motion that stays in motion.

EMBRACING YOUR BODY, BUM KNEE AND ALL

By the time we get to midlife, we all have our fair share of battle scars, and many of us are also nursing one kind of chronic injury or another. The truth is, although our muscles and ligaments tend to be pretty resilient, they are by no means indestructible. Couple that with some minor or major problems in the bones and joints, and it's inevitable that there are going to be some issues related to the normal wear and tear on your body.

Being a body in motion that stays in motion can be stressful. Whenever we get bumped from one state of velocity, and our momentum is changed, there are bound to be consequences. (See Newton's second law, the law of resultant force: A body in motion will stay in motion until it is acted upon by an outside force!)

As a physical therapist, I see all sorts of injuries that graphically illustrate Newton's second law. I see skiers recovering from blown-out anterior cruciate ligaments (a common knee injury when athletes engage in a sport where they have to start or stop very suddenly). Their stories are always very similar. "I was cruising along and I hit a patch of ice and . . ."

Truthfully, though, many of the injuries I see aren't sports related at all. I've had people who "stepped wrong" and tore the meniscus in their knees or people who, after years of running, suffer from chronic foot pain. And there are armies of people out there who suffer from back and shoulder problems because of sitting at a desk year after year after year.

We're all prone to injury. The big question is: How do we respond to it, in

THE BLESSING OF STRESSING

What is usually considered "normal wear and tear" on tissues in the body is actually the result of too much or too little physical stress to the involved area. This is true for ligaments, tendons, muscles, bones, and the cardiovascular system. Here's what research has shown about the effects of stress:

- Too little physical challenge and all tissues atrophy and weaken.

- Maintaining the same level of activity allows tissues to remain unchanged.

- Increase the challenge, and tissues respond: They get bigger, stronger, and more tolerant of physical stress.

- Too much stress and all tissues become inflamed, painful, or injured.

- Most Americans choose the "too little challenge" route. Exercise in the nursing home might entail simply having to lift the leg off the bed 10 times.

Cartilage, the resilient tissue that cushions your joints, also responds in a positive way to reasonable physical stress. With enough physical challenge, there is an increase in the amount of the shock-absorbing protein in cartilage called proteoglycans. But not all cartilage stress is beneficial. If you have excessive loading on a weight-bearing joint—such as the pressure on the knees if you're overweight—the cartilage that is damaged may not regenerate. And what happens to cartilage if a joint is not used at all? A study of paraplegics found that they had lost 25 percent of knee cartilage after 1 year in wheelchairs.

To keep all your tissues healthy, I advise you to avoid pain, maintain optimum weight, and regularly move your joints.

terms of maintaining (or improving) our current level of fitness? I'll guide you through that in the next part of this book, where I deal with specific joints and body parts and demonstrate how to work optimally with each. For now, let's get back to *getting up* and *getting out* of that chair—which might not be as easy as you think.

THE AIR SQUAT AND THE DOOR SQUAT

If you have trouble getting up out of a seat, you'll need to work on strengthening your leg muscles. This is relatively easy to do.

Here is an easy exercise that will get your thigh and butt muscles firing and will make getting up and down (hands free) a cinch. To do the *air squat*:

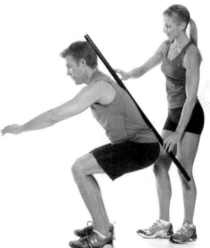

- Stand with your feet hip distance apart. Raise your arms out straight in front of you and lean forward. Keep your back straight.

- Now bend as though you were going to sit back into a chair. Watch your knees to make sure that they stay aligned over your feet and that they don't move "ahead" of your toes on the floor. Also, make sure your knees don't twist in or out, but stay exactly in line with your toes.

- Bend as low as you can go, pause, and then stand up. Keep your weight on your heels and lean forward.

Do this air squat at least six to eight times (that's a "set"). Build up to the point where you can repeat one set of six to eight air squats three times a day.

MAKING GRAVITY WORK FOR YOU

Of course, we all know what we're fighting against when we try to get up. It's called gravity. Gravity is what keeps us tethered to the ground. It's also the force that naturally offers our bodies resistance at all times, and resistance is a great builder of muscle and bone.

One of the things I ask guests at Canyon Ranch is: When was the last time

Another option is the *door squat*:

- Sit in a chair facing a door, with the open door between your legs but far enough away that you have to reach forward to grasp both knobs of the door handle.

- Use the doorknobs to help pull yourself up to a standing position.

- As you rise, do not allow your thighs to twist out of line with your toes.

When you stretch out your arms to reach the doorknobs, you automatically bring your whole body into alignment: your nose is over your toes, and your spine is straight. That's exactly the position you want to be in when you rise from a seat (with or without the assistance of door handles!). As you get stronger, focus on *not* relying on your arms to pull you forward.

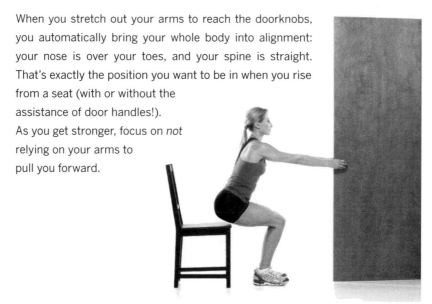

you were on the floor? Many people look at me dumbfounded. Unless guests have young children or grandchildren, most of them can't remember the last time they simply gave way to gravity and plunked themselves down on the floor. I ask my clients this, not as a clever way to prepare them for floor work in the gym, but to make an important point: One of the essential skills we all need to have for life is the ability to get ourselves up and off the floor.

(continued on page 26)

Dorothy's
STORY

One of my very first patients was a feisty 74-year-old woman named Dorothy. Dorothy was fiercely independent and lived in her own home with her cat. She decided she was going to put her house on the market and move into an apartment in an assisted-living community, just so that she wouldn't have to worry about long-term care when she eventually began to slow down. Her real estate agent suggested to Dorothy that refreshing the flower beds in her backyard would greatly increase her chances of a quick sale.

Dorothy had done a lot of gardening in the past, and she decided there was no reason she couldn't handle the whole garden renovation. She called a friend, who took her to the local nursery where they bought a couple pallets of flowering plants. Dorothy's friend helped her carry the pallets into her small, fenced-in backyard. But when he offered to help Dorothy with the planting, she shooed him away: "I've been a gardener all my life and I'll enjoy doing this myself."

(In fact, though, it had been several years since Dorothy had done any significant yard work; the most she did was turn on the tap for the sprinkler once a week.)

A couple of days later, Dorothy got around to the planting phase of her project. She put on her gardening gear, grabbed her old canvas gloves and a plastic knee pad, and got to work. At first, Dorothy was comfortable, kneeling on the pad and working way. But when she started to get up, she tripped, rolled off her knees (and the cushion), and slumped to her side. Both knees, she realized, were hurting her terribly. She rubbed them, trying to make the pain go away. A few minutes later, when she tried to get to her feet, she found she couldn't. The harder she tried, the more frightened she became.

She was just too weak to get up. Her problem wasn't knee pain, but just an inability to get up from the ground without climbing up on furniture (which wasn't in the garden).

Dorothy was too embarrassed to shout for help. She actually sat in her garden—hungry, thirsty, and quite sore—through the following day and night. It was the morning of the second day before she heard her neighbor's back door open. She called out for help and, fortunately, her neighbor heard her. I met her that afternoon in the hospital.

When I interviewed Dorothy, she was resting comfortably and was being given fluids intravenously. She hadn't suffered any broken bones, but, on examination, I found her to be quite weak in her legs and trunk. She couldn't kneel without falling over because the muscles in her trunk were too weak.

I asked Dorothy to describe her lifestyle to me.

"Well," she began, "I've always considered myself pretty healthy. I take care of my own home, do my own laundry, and prepare my own meals. I volunteer once a week at a local hospital, and I drive all over town."

Then I asked her a question that startled her: "Do you have a bathtub in your home?"

"Why, no, I don't. Only a shower."

"Well, do you climb stairs?"

"Truthfully? Not often," she said. "That's one of the benefits of living in a single-level house."

And finally I asked her, "When was the last time you got down on the floor?"

At this she laughed and said, "Does last night count?"

Dorothy was actually really lucky in more ways than one. Had her neighbor been out of town, she may have suffered some serious consequences of exposure—or worse. And she hadn't broken a bone, which meant she could start physical therapy right away.

All the exercises she did at first made use of the simple, universal resistance device I have already mentioned—gravity. Gravity's natural resistance helps build muscles and bone strength, simply by using body weight. It was important for Dorothy to learn how to use gravity to her advantage—so that it wouldn't work against her ever again.

The simple task of getting off the floor pretty much activates every muscle and joint in our bodies. First we get onto our hands and knees, and then push ourselves up using our hands, wrists, and arms. We bend at the waist, tilt our neck and head, bend our knees, and move our feet. If someone can get down on the floor and then get up easily, that person is actually in pretty good condition.

Being in Balance

Many people, especially those who are a bit older, have some balance issues. Some are caused by health problems, others by medication. No matter what the cause, everyone's balance can be improved, and this is really important if you are to embark on a fitness program with as much openness and preparedness as possible.

One of the first things I do with guests at the Ranch is to challenge their balance. I make them walk a "tightrope." Not literally, of course, but close enough. The "rope" they have to walk is a piece of foam about 6 inches wide, which I lay on the floor to form a single, straight, narrow path for about 10 feet. This is the tightrope they have to walk, carefully placing one foot in front of the other, without "falling off" to left or right. To add a bit of fun, I sometimes put a plastic alligator on the floor next to the "tightrope."

As guests make their way across the rope, many of them scream and flail their arms when they "fall into the drink." It sounds silly, and it is. But it works. We repeat the tightrope walk daily, and by the end of a week their balance has improved.

It's simple enough to try this tightrope challenge on your own turf if you want to. Walk heel to toe; imagine you *are* on a tightrope, and practice walking in a very straight line, one foot directly in front of another.

In addition, here are some other simple things you can do at home to improve your balance:

○ Do some safe, routine tasks, such as brushing your teeth, with your eyes closed. (Sounds simple, but with your eyes closed, only gravity helps determine your balance; all the visual cues are missing.)

○ If you're standing in line, lift one leg and bend it at the knee. Stand on the other leg, with your hands at your sides, for as long as possible. If this seems too easy, do the same thing with your eyes closed.

○ Practice standing on one foot while slowly turning your head left and right.

○ Practice walking in slow motion on uneven or soft surfaces.

FINDING YOUR MOTIVATION

Often, we need some kind of wake-up call to get active, but after that, even when we're in a pattern of regular daily movement, we may slide into another pattern of not doing much at all.

If you're anything like me, the falloff in regular exercise usually goes something like this. If I miss a day of activity during a week, no sweat. But if I miss two, then I need to refocus. And if I end up missing three, it's usually a sign that I'm getting way off track and I have to haul my body—and motivation—back into the picture.

That's why I want to offer you, at the outset, some simple things you can do to get and stay motivated:

○ Tape up a picture of yourself at your most fit and healthy where you'll see it every day, such as next to the bathroom mirror.

○ Post motivating notes around your house, such as "You are one workout away from feeling better."

○ Treat yourself to the purchase of a good pair of running shoes and wear them as often as possible.

○ Hang a picture of your fitness role model on your fridge (could be a professional athlete, but could also be your great aunt who just came back from a trek to the Great Wall of China at the age of 85).

○ Socialize with others who are committed to improving their level of fitness.

Whatever you need to do to bolster your motivation—do it. Every time you take another step, try a new activity, and in any way improve your strength, flexibility, and endurance, you'll be keeping yourself prime for life.

CHAPTER THREE

FLEXIBILITY

"Stay committed to your decisions, but
stay flexible in your approach."
—*Tom Robbins*

"Therefore the stiff and unbending is the
disciple of death. The gentle and yielding
is the disciple of life."
—*Lao Tsu,* **Tao Te Ching**

Let yourself go back in time and visualize what playing really felt like when you
were a child. Remember clambering all over the jungle gym? Or the soaring
feeling you'd get on a swing? Or do you remember playing hide-and-seek and
finding a ridiculously difficult place to hide, where you'd have to scrunch up and
contort your body in impossible ways?

Some of us were freakishly flexible. When I was a kid, the real contortionists
were what we called "double-jointed." We'd show off to our friends by bending
our hands backward or doing a crazy split. Others of us were less flexible, but
strong: We could hit the ball the farthest, or we became the youngest player to
make the varsity team in some sport.

The point is, we all started out, as children, with different levels of strength and flexibility. Those differences become more pronounced and noticeable as we age. Though you might think super-flexible people are the ones least likely to get injured, the opposite is the case. Those who are super-flexible, with longer, looser muscles and joints, are more prone to injury. Those who have shorter and stronger muscles may not be able to touch their toes (and this is fine!) but perhaps can still ski the "diamond" slopes with less fear of injury.

For some reason, a lot of people have a misconception about what flexibility is, why it's important, and what level of flexibility we ought to strive for. There is actually a lot of confusing and contradictory information pumped into the mainstream by well-meaning fitness and health pros. Too often, we think of those who exhibit extreme flexibility as somehow being "fitter" or "healthier" than the rest of us. Maybe it's because this kind of movement is so dramatic. (Think of the amazing performers in Cirque du Soleil or the incredible gymnasts in Olympic competition.) But it's not so. The fact is, extreme flexibility, from the perspective of joint and muscle health, can actually be a *liability*: It can actually make one prone to *more* injury.

More often than not, this confusion arises because terms are misused.

To get the first misconception out of the way, flexibility is not synonymous with fitness. The fact that you can do a split does *not* mean you are more fit than someone who cannot do one! So I hope you'll come away from this chapter with a fresh understanding of what it means to be adequately flexible, then use this information to maximize your level of fitness.

WHAT KIND OF FLEXIBILITY DO YOU REALLY NEED?

For starters, I want to help you make the distinction—in your own experience and in your own body—between desirable flexibility, the kind you need for life-long mobility, and *hyper*-flexibility, the kind that can cause lasting injury. Most of us don't need to get anywhere near the flexibility of gymnasts, contortionists, trapeze artists, or certain yoga masters. In fact, it's not even desirable. What most of us need to work on, instead, is range of motion. The goal, for most of us, is not

A LESSON LEARNED . . . THE HARD WAY

When I was much younger, I held the view shared by so many physical fitness enthusiasts—that there was something extra-special about being extra-flexible. In fact, I was quite competitive about it—until I learned better.

My comeuppance occurred when I was teaching an aerobics and stretching class at a local gym. During one particular class, I noticed a woman who was obviously quite proud of her flexibility. While I led the class in a gentle version of a forward split—where you rest on one knee and slide the other leg out in front of you as far as comfortably possible—this woman dropped down and slid her leg all the way out. Then she looked at me with a slightly superior smile on her face. Not to be outdone, I dropped into my own full split and grinned back at her.

The next stretch was a classic. I had everyone sit on the floor, spreading his or her legs in a wide "V," and lean forward. I asked them to keep their spines straight and to take this stretch only to the *very edge* of discomfort. For most people, this means being able to tilt slightly forward, usually no more than a 45-degree angle. This woman, however, was able to lean all the way forward, with her chest touching the floor. From that position she looked up at me as though to say, "Try topping this!" And so I did. The war was on.

After that, we moved through a series of stretches until I found one that she couldn't quite master. As the class ended I felt triumphant.

Not for long! The next day—more truthfully, for days after that—I paid for this vanity: I walked around like a crippled old man, even though I was in my twenties. I had actually pulled both groin muscles! And I had only myself to blame. I had completely disregarded my own hyper-flexibility and needlessly injured myself.

It was probably that experience that prompted me to begin to study movement—and especially flexibility—much more closely.

the ability to be remarkably flexible but the ability to attain, and retain, the greatest mobility possible.

Having optimum flexibility means that you have good range of motion in your joints. That range of motion is easily and—this is really important—*painlessly* attained. In other words, flexibility is specific to a particular joint or series of joints. Very few people are just "flexible" as a body type. In fact, someone can be flexible in one way with a joint and not in another. (That splitter? She may be able to do a front split, but not a side split.)

So you may be quite flexible in one joint and not in another. And this is where a "weekend warrior"—someone who exercises hard but only occasionally—can get into trouble. If you don't properly condition yourself, the joints that haven't been getting much use can be seriously injured. And it can happen fast.

When we think of someone as being "inflexible," in truth, she might be as flexible as she needs to be. For instance, consider the octogenarian who may need a walker for balance but is perfectly capable of reaching up to take a can from the top kitchen shelf. Or the weight lifter who can bench-press 500 pounds but who can't touch his toes. These people are not experiencing a loss of a range of motion; on the contrary, they're using their range of motion (flexibility) wisely.

When someone is truly experiencing a lack of flexibility, what he's dealing with is a *limited* range of motion. This can happen because of injury or lack of use. The goal when someone comes to me for treatment of inflexibility is to restore that person's range of motion to the appropriate level—not to push that person's joints and ligaments beyond what they're best suited for. This is the part of flexibility that people seem to lose sight of: It's all about appropriateness—not extremes.

Another way to think about flexibility is to think of it in terms of mobility. A limited range of motion, a loss of flexibility, means less mobility. As we age, we tend to lose some range of motion unless we stretch to maintain it.

WHAT IS ADEQUATE RANGE OF MOTION?

Having an adequate range of motion all depends on your needs. A swimmer needs loose shoulders and feet in the water. A dancer needs flexible hamstrings to help perform ballet.

Runners and walkers who have stiffer lower extremities (improved by range of motion exercises) were found to run with more energy economy: Their stiffer tissues store energy to help them rebound and push off on the next step.

WARMING UP VERSUS STRETCHING

At Canyon Ranch, we tend to encourage people to warm up before an activity and to save the stretching for later. Research shows that pre-stretching does not reduce the risk of injury, which is contrary to popular belief.

Warming up entails increasing body temperature. For example, if you're going to embark on a brisk walk, start slowly and gradually increase the speed. At Canyon Ranch, this has been our policy for many years, and it is one reason we have a wonderful safety record.

Let me say it again: Start slowly, and increase gradually.

If you are doing an activity that requires range of motion such as dance, the same thing applies. But when you are warmed up, don't start kicking those legs up high immediately. Progressively increase range of motion, or gently move joints in gentle circular motions to get the juices flowing. Then, at the end of the session, you can stretch and work on flexibility. That carries over into the next workout.

If you've been relatively inactive for a long time, and you're just getting into a program to develop flexibility, you need to be careful about what you try, and make sure you're helping your joints and not hurting them. The movements illustrated and described in this chapter are not "just" exercises. Every movement that you make—whether stretching, flexing, or warming up—helps your body perform in new ways. As anyone who has tried yoga or tai chi knows, your mood and your body are transformed when you work on flexibility carefully and correctly.

Among the flexing, stretching, relaxing, and range of motion exercises that I describe in this chapter, many are designed to address specific parts of the body—from the latissimus dorsi, pectoralis, and spine to the gastrocnemius, soleus, and hamstring (all of which I'll explain). However "targeted" my recommendations are, your whole body will benefit. Every one of these exercises will prepare you for being prime for life.

ARE YOU HYPERMOBILE?

Some people, as mentioned, are what we call hypermobile. Since I'm among them, I'm quite aware of the extra risks that come with the hand we've been dealt.

A flexible body certainly has its benefits. But it can also have its drawbacks. A football lineman about to be hit on the side of his knee by another 250-pound behemoth needs joint stability and adequate range of motion for each joint—but he doesn't need flexibility in his knees, that's for sure. In fact, a highly flexible joint is just what he *doesn't* need because it's more unstable. A stiff knee, for example, literally locks into its most stable position when straight. A hypermobile one is much more prone to damage.

How does anyone tell the difference? Often you can tell just by looking. If someone stands up straight and his or her knees bow out behind the body (that's called a "negative range of degree"), it means the joint is hyperextended. That person has knees that are much more prone to damage than someone who has normal knee flexibility.

Awareness is growing—among biomechanists and physical therapists—that we're all beginning to understand that there is no benefit to working a muscle or ligament beyond its adequate range of motion. In addition, research is showing that people with hypermobile joints may be at greater risk of osteoarthritis—the kind of arthritis (commonly called "age related") that occurs when there's joint deterioration.

Our bodies are pretty good communicators when it comes to indicating our level of flexibility. That's why some of us are naturally drawn to activities that require flexibility, such as yoga or swimming, while others are more comfortable with contact sports, where flexibility is more a deficit than an asset. But sometimes, we don't quite listen to our bodies.

The Beighton Index Test

What follows is a test you can use to find out just how flexible you already are. Just be sure, as you follow these directions, that you don't strain yourself. Stop immediately if you experience any pain.

You can take the Beighton Index test at home. Although you can do some of these evaluations alone, you'll need to ask a friend or partner to help you with others.

○ Take off your shoes and stand up straight with your feet hip distance apart. Keep your knees straight. Bend at the hips and try to place the palms of your hands flat on the floor. If you can do this, give yourself one point.

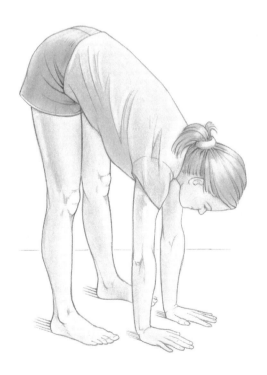

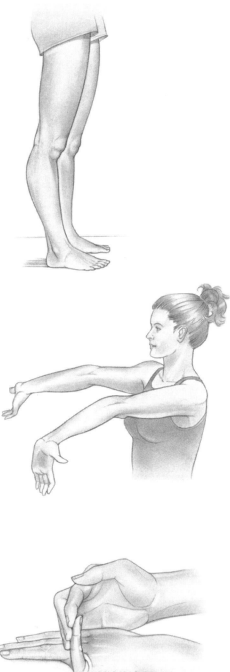

○ Stand and lock your knees. Have your friend watch from the side and notice whether your knees go beyond straight and bow back noticeably (hyperextend). If this happens, give yourself one point for each knee that bows back.

○ Reach your arms out to your sides, palms up. Straighten and lock your elbows. If they go beyond straight to backward, you get one point for each elbow.

○ Place the palm of your hand and forearm down on a table. Can you easily bend your little finger back and up to 90 degrees? You get one point for each little finger bending backward.

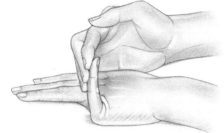

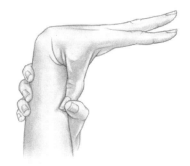

○ Can you easily bend your thumb down to your wrist? You get one point for each thumb that bends to your wrist.

Add up your points. If you scored four or more, you are considered hypermobile. This is a pretty informal test, but it will give you an idea of your level of joint flexibility. If you scored more than four and you have preexisting joint pain, it might be time to see a physical therapist or talk to your doctor.

What can you learn from this test? Here's an example of someone I worked with who took the test and subsequently changed her approach to movement.

Marjorie's
STORY

Marjorie was a yoga teacher. She came to me because she felt limited in the poses she could do and she complained about feeling "tight." I went to watch her teach a yoga class to get a sense of what she meant. She knew every posture well and demonstrated excellent alignment. I also noticed that each pose she chose to do was one that really challenged the range of motion of her joints. She included very few postures that worked on strength and stability.

When we got together afterward, Marjorie told me she had been drawn to yoga because it had helped her "become more flexible." This comment intrigued me, and I asked her if I could give her the Beighton Index test in order to test her for hypermobility. Being a good sport, she agreed.

Marjorie scored a nine on the Beighton Index, which showed that she had always been flexible—even hyper-flexible. I suggested that she add postures to her repertoire that would balance her hypermobility with strengthening and stabilizing her joints. I added that she just might feel more "flexible" as a result.

She looked at me, a bit confused. She didn't understand how my recommendations for strengthening and stabilizing would, in fact, help her out.

I reminded her that her hyper-flexibility was actually preventing her from doing a number of postures she'd be able to do if she worked on strength and stability. "And," I added, "when you can do a wider range of things, doesn't that mean you are more flexible?"

I think a lightbulb went off in her head at that moment. She smiled and agreed.

TO KNOW YOUR BODY, TEST IT

The following stretches are designed to help you test your range of motion and find out whether you need to do some stretching to increase joint flexibility and avoid injury during exercise. Before you start experimenting with the stretches, however, I want to remind you: *Pain is not okay!* If you have any pain, discontinue and see a physical therapist.

Here are some simplified self-tests that may give you an idea of a few problems you may experience in different areas. When you learn to take care of them, your activity level will soar.

Upper Trapezius Test

Look in the mirror. Do your shoulders slope significantly downward from your neck and do you have a history of headaches, or neck or shoulder pain? If this is you, stop stretching your upper trapezius and the side of your neck. See the shoulder chapter and the neck chapter for detailed help.

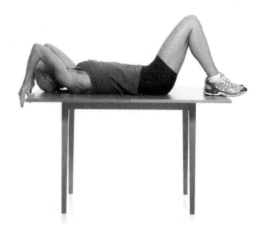

Latissimus Dorsi Test

Lie on your bed or on a table on your back, with your knees bent. Bend your elbows and keep your forearms parallel to one another. Slowly raise your arms over your head. Try to rest the backs of your upper arms on the bed or table. If you can't bring your arms within a few inches of the bed or table, you may need the **latissimus dorsi stretch (page 45)**.

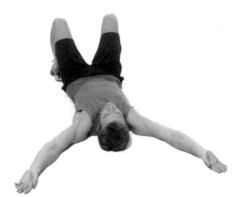

Pectoralis Major Test

Lie on your back with your knees bent, feet flat. Keeping your lower back down but relaxed, reach up diagonally and out with both arms, palms up. Keep your elbows straight and lower your arms to the floor or bed. If you can't reach the surface with the backs of your elbows, forearms, and hands, you need the **pectoralis major stretch (page 46)**. Few people have truly short pectoralis major muscles.

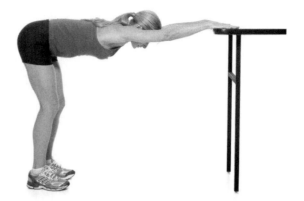

Thoracic Spine/Pelvic Control Test

Place your hands on the edge of a kitchen counter and step back until you can bend at the waist and your back is at a 90-degree angle to the floor (you will look like a table). Allow your knees to bend slightly, so you don't feel much of a stretch in your hamstrings or the backs of your thighs. Slowly lower your shoulders. If this causes you discomfort, you may have a stiff upper back (thoracic spine). Add the **quadruped rock back (page 48)** and **"L" stretch (page 47)** to your repertoire.

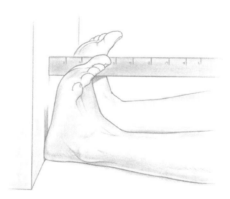

Gastrocnemius Test

Sit down with your legs outstretched and your heels lightly against a wall. Lean back so that your hamstrings aren't getting any stretch. Keeping your knees down, can you "dorsiflex," or pull the ball of your feet an inch off of the wall? If not, add the **gastrocnemius stretch (page 50)** to your new routine.

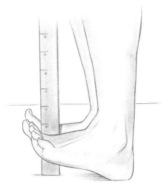

Soleus Test

Sit on a straight-backed chair. Slide forward on the chair until your knees are at a right angle (90 degrees). Try to lift your forefeet off the floor, keeping your heels down. If you can't lift the ball of your foot off the floor 1 inch, add the **soleus stretch (page 51)** to your routine.

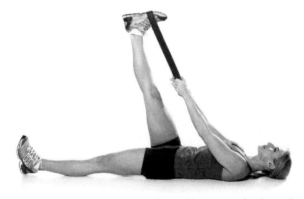

Hamstrings Test

Lie on your back and draw one leg up as high as comfort allows, with the other leg extended along the floor in front of you. Make sure you keep your lower back and tailbone on the floor. If your leg is about 80 degrees up off the floor, your hamstring range is excellent. If it is 90 or more, you may be too flexible. If it is 70 degrees or less, you need the **hamstring stretch (page 52)**. If this causes you any severe pain almost as soon as you lift your leg, or you have pain down the back of your thigh, it can indicate a lower back problem. Pain felt in the hip or front of the groin can be indicative of what's called an acetabular labral tear. You should see your doctor or a physical therapist if you have pain in either of these areas.

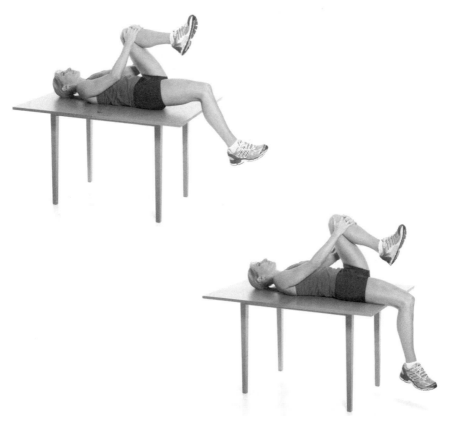

Hip Flexors Test

Lie on your back on a firm bed or on a table with your hips about 8 to 10 inches from the edge. With your hands, pull the left thigh toward your chest just enough to lightly press your lower back down. Slowly lower your right leg over the edge of the table or bed and relax it down. Your right knee should be a few inches out over the edge of the table or bed. Don't let your right thigh drift out to the side. If the back of your right thigh is not down on the bed, or your knee is bent at more than 100 degrees, or both, you need to add the **quadriceps stretch (page 53)** and **hip flexor stretch (page 54)** to your routine. Be sure to keep your right foot pointing straight ahead. If it can't, or if you have knee pain, you may have a short/stiff iliotibial band. If you have lower back pain, try the hip flexor stretch gently. If it exacerbates lower back pain, see a doctor or a physical therapist.

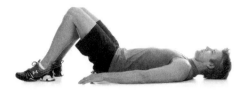

Neck Test *(You will need a friend or partner to help you with this one)*

Lie on your back, on the floor. Tuck your chin in and then gently press the back of your neck down toward the floor. If you can't get your forehead slightly higher than your chin, you have "forward head" position, which indicates that the superficial front neck muscles are too short. This can contribute to neck pain and headaches. If your neck easily does this *and* you have neck pain, you may have cervical flexion syndrome (see Chapter 9).

STRETCHES I DO NOT RECOMMEND

● Those that increase flexibility of the lower back. Research shows that most lower back problems are caused by excessive motion in the lower back combined with inadequate stability. Forget the lower back twists and extreme forward bends, especially if you have a history of lower back pain.

● Splits and stretches that hyperextend the hip. They decrease stability and integrity of the joint. Being able to perform splits or put your ankles around your neck may be a good party trick, but in the long run it's better for your orthopedic surgeon than for you.

● Stretches that forcibly put your arm behind your back. This sort of stretch may overstress the front of your shoulder capsule, so don't do it if you have any shoulder pain.

Physical therapists work hard at perfecting these tests and interpreting the results accurately. For a truly comprehensive posture and musculoskeletal evaluation, see an expert who does this all the time. These tests will give you some idea of potential problem areas and allow you to begin addressing them.

THE STRETCHES

As I've mentioned previously, I don't recommend stretching *before* you exercise. However, it is okay to stretch afterward or at other times during the day. Within reason, all of us can benefit from some stretching, but some of us need to be very gentle with it.

Most people can do all the following stretches after a workout. Even if you're very flexible, you can do them all very gently for a short time (not trying to progress farther into each). Those who discover "problem areas" are encouraged to do them frequently two to four times a day for 20 to 30 seconds each, repeating twice (if possible).

How to Stretch

Stretching is relaxing, and it is also a way of teaching ourselves patience. Stretching is a form of coaxing, a gentle reminder to muscles, ligaments, and tendons that they're designed to expand and contract. If you try to force a stretch, your body will rebel, and you will know it. (I don't do much stretching myself, except in my problem areas.)

The goal of stretching is to care for our joints so that they can function at their full range of motion. When you stretch, work to push to the edge of discomfort—but not into it. Stretching should be something you can do while breathing slowly and mindfully.

With the right kind of patience and focus, we can actually feel our muscles relax. (You will notice that when you exhale, your muscles tend to relax just a little. Use that to gently advance into each stretch a little more.)

How much stretching do you need?

If you scored greater than four on the Beighton Index test, I recommend that you don't stretch aggressively. Keep it very gentle. Avoid allowing those joints to hyperextend. Avoid all discomfort, and don't progress into each stretch (that's especially true if you're using the joints you discovered were hypermobile).

Perform each stretch for at least 30 seconds, gently stretching farther if you have no discomfort. For especially stiff, short muscles, repeat these stretches several times. Doing them two to four times a day is best. Remember, stop if you experience any pain or discomfort. (They also make a nice postexercise stretching routine.)

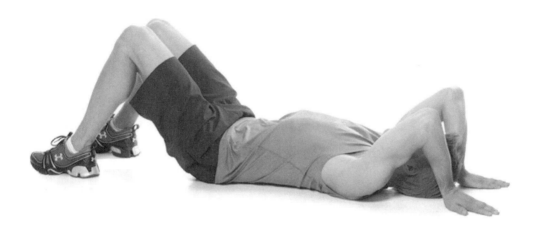

LATISSIMUS DORSI STRETCH

This is like the latissimus dorsi test, except you can do this on the floor. Lie on your back, with your knees bent. Keeping your elbows bent and your forearms parallel, slowly reach back over your head with your hands. Place your hands palms down on the floor with your fingers pointing back and your thumbs on the outside.

Keeping your upper arms parallel and your palms down, slide your hands back on the floor until you feel a stretch under your arm and shoulder region. Keep your elbows pointed up, not out. If you feel any discomfort on top of your shoulder, you are trying too hard. Keep it gentle, and over the next few weeks, you'll find that you will be able to slide your arms farther and farther back, without discomfort. Short, stiff latissimus dorsi cause the spine to round, and push the neck and temporomandibular joint in the jaw out of alignment. They are a major cause of shoulder problems.

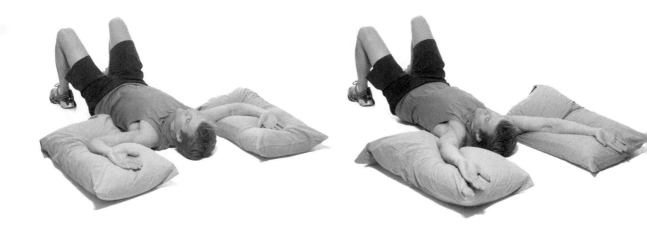

PECTORALIS MAJOR STRETCH

Lie on your back on the floor. Bend your elbows at a right angle and swing them out to your side so that your forearms are on the floor with your palms facing the ceiling and your elbows out straight from your shoulders. If you can't get comfortable in this position on the floor, place pillows beside you, and rest your arms on them.

Press your elbows and forearms down into the pillows firmly. You should feel a stretch across the chest and the middle trapezius muscle across the middle of your back working hard. Slowly slide your forearms toward your ears as far as comfort allows. Stop immediately if you encounter pain anywhere in the chest or shoulder. Linger at each point of stretch for 10 to 20 seconds. Spend a minute or two for this stretch as often as you can. This stretches the pectoralis major muscles, the medial rotators of the shoulders, and strengthens the middle trapezius muscles in the upper back. It is an excellent stretch to improve posture and prevent shoulder problems. Many people mistakenly pull their shoulders back by squeezing the shoulder blades together using the rhomboids. Doing so narrows and drops the shoulders and contributes to neck and shoulder problems. This exercise gives your chest openness, which will ease the strain on your shoulders. As you become more flexible, diminish the height of the pillows (or folded towels), until you can perform the entire stretch flat on the floor without any support.

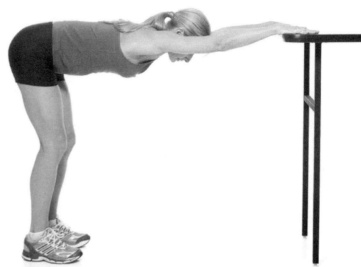

THE "L" STRETCH

Place your hands on the edge of a kitchen counter, shoulder width apart. Step back, lowering your upper body until you are as close to a right angle as comfort allows and your heels are directly below your buttocks. Keep your elbows straight. Begin with knees bent and try to point your "sitting bones" (i.e., your buttocks) up toward the ceiling. You are trying to create a flat back, not trying to arch your lower back.

If you have a flexible lower back, feel discomfort there, or have a big arch, keep your belly pulled in (or brace your midsection—see Chapter 9) to prevent your lower back from hurting or arching too much. Focus on gently flattening the upper back. As you exhale, gently let your upper back sink. Keep your neck in line with the rest of your spine.

Tall people will get a stronger stretch, so they may need to simply lift the upper body up a bit higher. Experiment with tucking your tailbone under and tilting it up—all gently. If you learn to use the muscles controlling your pelvis, that will also be helpful in controlling your back. Keep it gentle and soothing. Remember, any stretch you hate is one you are probably forcing.

To include the hamstrings in this stretch, gently straighten your knees enough to stretch the muscles in back of your thighs. That will stretch the hamstrings. Don't force it, and if you found you have hyperextended knees, do not lock them! Hold this stretch for up to a minute. Repeat frequently throughout the day. This stretches the entire back of your body—the erector spinae, latissimus dorsi, triceps, pectoralis major, hamstrings, and gastrocnemius. Humans tend to become more rounded over with age. This helps you remain your tallest.

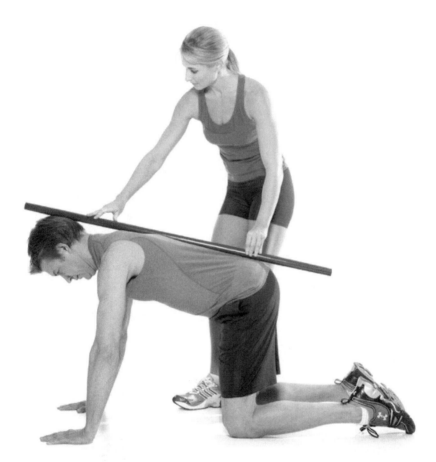

QUADRUPED ROCK BACK STRETCH

Get on your hands and knees on a padded surface. Push back with your hands, rocking your hips back. Do not sit back using your hip muscles. Instead, push yourself slowly back with straight arms, keeping your spine straight. Think of aiming your buttocks to the ceiling with your spine straight. If you feel any discomfort in your lower back or shoulders, it is because you are *sitting* back, using your hip flexors rather than your serratus anterior muscles. These muscles are important shoulder muscles—they rotate the shoulder blades upward. Keep the back of your neck elongated. Do not drop your head down or lift it up.

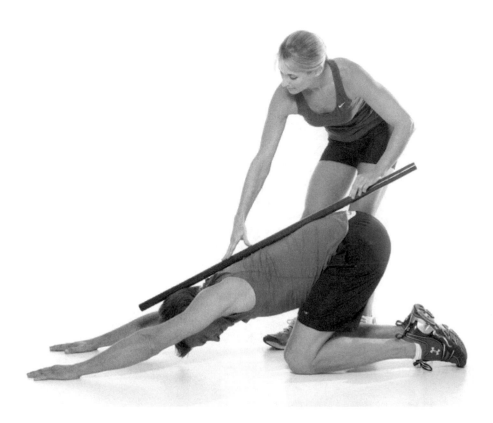

Allow your shoulders to rise up naturally toward your ears, but don't *force* them up. This exercise activates the serratus anterior, gently decreases any rotation or abnormal bending in the spine, and improves flexibility of the hip extensors such as the gluteus maximus. It also gently stretches a lower back that excessively extends. Although subtle, it may be the most powerful stretch we are doing. It can reverse many shoulder, neck, middle back, hip, and lower back problems. If it doesn't, you are not doing it properly or are trying to go too far into it. Unlike the others, repeat this one five to 10 times.

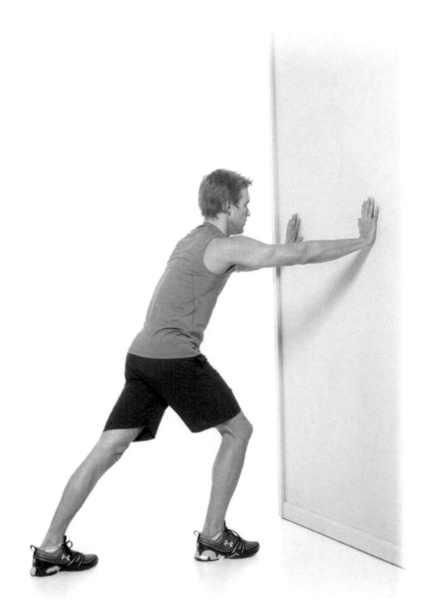

GASTROCNEMIUS STRETCH

Stand up straight and place your hands against a wall or countertop. Slide your left foot back as far as you can with your heel flat on the floor and your left foot straight ahead. Keeping the left knee straight and your heel down, gently bend the right knee forward until you feel a gentle, painless stretch in your left upper calf. Gently hold this for 30 to 60 seconds, then switch feet and repeat on the other leg. This stretches the gastrocnemius and plantaris muscles in the calf. Make sure your foot stays flat on the floor and doesn't roll in or out. Keep the arch lifted. Repeat on both sides.

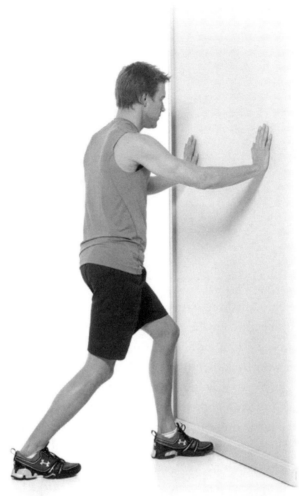

SOLEUS STRETCH

Press your hands against a wall or the edge of a countertop. Slide your left foot back, but not as far as you did with the gastrocnemius stretch. Keeping your left heel down, gently bend your left knee until you feel a stretch in the left calf and/or Achilles tendon region. Gently hold for 30 to 60 seconds. Change position, bringing your left foot forward and right foot back. This stretches the soleus muscle in the calf. It is important to stretch both the gastrocnemius and the soleus muscles. A disparity of length may lead to Achilles tendon problems. Again, don't allow your ankles or feet to move out of alignment. Avoid allowing the foot to roll in or out. Keep the arch lifted.

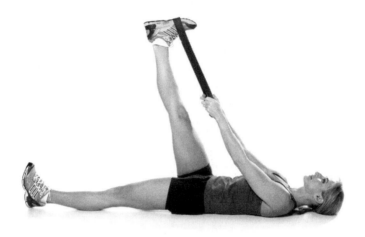

HAMSTRING STRETCH

This stretches all three hamstring muscles. For activities such as running, the hamstrings need adequate length to function well.

You'll need a strap or belt for this stretch.

Lie on your back, bending both knees, feet flat on the floor. Take a belt long enough (double your height, just to be certain it is long enough) so that you can loop it around your foot to control your foot with your hands and keep your shoulders on the floor and place the center of it around the arch of your right foot. Lift the leg, and as you do so, use the belt to lift your right foot up toward the ceiling very slowly. Keep your knee slightly bent as the foot rises. Bring the right thigh and leg up just enough to feel a slight stretch in the back of the thigh. Gently rotate your leg and foot in and out to find the angle that feels most restricted. Focus on that angle—gently.

Allow your toes to point up so you don't limit the stretch to the gastrocnemius muscle. Focus on keeping your lower back and tailbone down. Find your point of slight stretch and progress gently.

If your leg is straight up and your tailbone is down, you may have excessive flexibility in your hamstrings, which may cause some weakness. Pain radiating down your thigh into the calf and foot may indicate sciatic nerve involvement. Stop doing this stretch immediately and consult a physical therapist if you experience this.

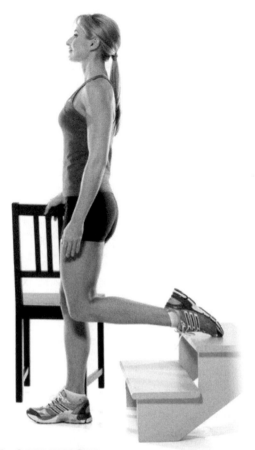

QUADRICEPS STRETCH (*focusing on the rectus femoris muscle*)

Stand with your back turned to a step. With your right hand, use the wall or a chair for support. With the left, lift your left foot, and put your left foot back on a stair or the seat of the chair. (Lift with your hand—don't bring your foot up to your hand or to the stair. This may cause a cramp.) Your foot should be back far enough so that your bent knee is behind the foot you're standing on. Stand up straight, with your weight-bearing knee slightly bent. Tighten your buttocks and brace your midsection. You should feel a gentle stretch in the front of your thigh up to your groin.

To increase the stretch, bend your standing knee a bit more, pushing your foot farther back on the step or chair. The higher the step upon which you place the foot, the stronger the stretch. You are stretching the four quadriceps, with a focus on the most troublesome one—the rectus femoris. This muscle flexes the hips, so it affects the knee, hips, and lower back if too short. If you feel any lower back discomfort with this stretch, you have not braced properly and your lower back is not in a safe, neutral position.

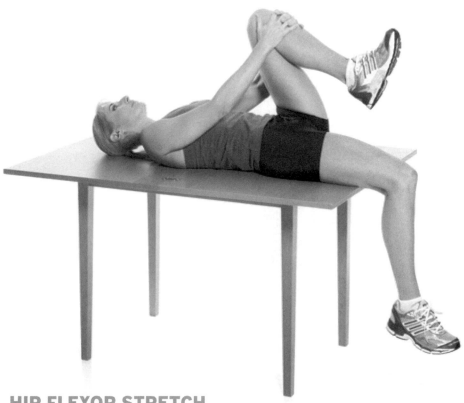

HIP FLEXOR STRETCH

Lie on your back on a firm bed or table with your hips 8 to 10 inches from the edge. Start with both feet up on the edge or hold them both. Pull one thigh into your chest just enough to press your lower back down lightly. Do not allow your lower back or buttocks to roll up off the bed. Slowly lower your other leg over the edge, easing it down. The knee will need to be a few inches from the edge of the bed. Don't let it wander out to the side.

You should feel a stretch in the groin and, slightly, in the small of your lower back. The iliacus, rectus femoris, and psoas muscles are being stretched. A too-short psoas is a major contributor to lower back pain in some people—pulling them into an arched lower back. If you have lower back pain, try the hip flexor stretch gently. If it makes lower back pain worse, see a physical therapist. If your iliotibial band is too short or stiff and your foot on the dropped leg tends to turn out, turn it in just enough to feel a stretch in the outer thigh without knee pain. If you feel knee pain when you're doing this, experiment with turning your foot in or out enough to avoid any pain.

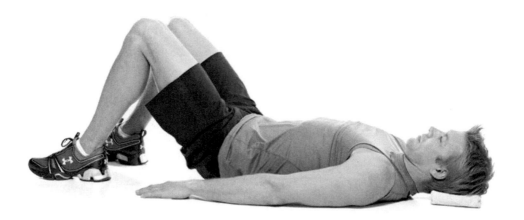

NECK STRETCH

Lie on your back on the floor, looking straight up, with your head aligned with your spine. Tuck in your chin and gently press the back of your neck down into the floor. If you can't get your forehead slightly higher than your chin, put a small, rolled hand towel under the back of your head so that your forehead is slightly higher than your chin. Tuck in your chin again and try to lengthen the back of your neck into the floor, in a nodding motion.

You should not be able to touch your neck to the floor, because the neck should curve slightly up and away from the floor. If your entire neck does touch the floor, don't do this stretch. It won't benefit you and could overstretch the neck the wrong way. You should feel a stretch in the front, beside your throat on either side, and along the back of your neck. Hold for 10 seconds. Repeat five to 10 times. This stretches the scalenes that pull your neck forward and also strengthens the deep neck flexors in the front of your neck. It can reverse forward head posture and help relieve some chronic headaches. If pain occurs in your neck or down the arms, stop immediately.

CHAPTER FOUR

MUSCLE STRENGTH

"Activity of the nervous system improves
the capacity for activity, just as exercising a
muscle makes it stronger."

—*Dr. Ralph Gerard*

"First we inspire them,
then we perspire them."

—*Jack LaLanne, the Godfather of Fitness*

Someone recently asked me what Jack LaLanne is up to these days. I admit, I had to do a bit of digging around, but it seems that he's doing what he's done for the past 50 years—and then some. He still works tirelessly to inspire people the world over to get up and get moving through books, radio programs, videos, exercise equipment, nutritional information, and products—you name it. In 1976, at the age of 62, Jack LaLanne commemorated the "Spirit of '76" by swimming 1 mile in Long Beach Harbor, handcuffed, shackled, and towing 13 boats—representing the 13 original colonies—and containing 76 people. He is still going strong today at age 94. I included his famous remark "People don't die of old age, they die of inactivity" as an epigraph to this book, because if anyone has proven this to be true, it would be Mr. LaLanne.

If we are to give in to the vicissitudes of life and slow down, then yes, our muscle strength will wane as we age, but this doesn't have to happen. Our muscles can be increased and strengthened throughout our lifetimes; we just need to make the commitment to being active, and, especially, to building our strength.

When we talk about strength, what we're referring to is the muscle's ability to exert force. (By the way, strength and resistance training are one and the same thing.) Whether you're a seasoned athlete or an occasional Sunday golfer, you can build and maintain your muscle strength every day.

STRENGTH-BUILDING ACTIVITIES

If you think about it for a moment, you'll see that you have opportunities all day long to build up your strength, even if you don't know it. When you rearranged your living room furniture, you were strength-training. Whenever you shop at one of the big box retailers and buy items in bulk (especially laundry detergent) and lug it to your car, you are strength-training. Unfortunately, we don't lift and carry a 20-pound box of detergent every day, so most of us need to make a concerted effort and establish a regular strength-training program. That's where I can be of help.

Countless studies have shown us that when people increase their strength, their risk factors for conditions that we consider to be normal parts of aging disappear or decrease dramatically. All we have to do is look at the elderly in other cultures to see how true this is. In many countries, older people still work alongside the young and they are still vital family members, participating in all of the (strength-training) tasks of everyday life.

For some reason, in our country, we've always thought about our later years as the time to slow down, if not stop; we've actually been encouraged to "retire" from life. Thank God that way of thinking has finally changed. Just because we reach a certain chronological age doesn't mean we shouldn't be able to lift a bag of groceries, lift the mattress when we change a bed, or twist that cap off a jar of pickles.

When you engage in strength-building activities, you prime your body in so many ways, including increasing its metabolic (fat-burning) rate, building and maintaining bone density (so forestalling the onset of osteoporosis), keeping your brain well primed and functioning (and your mood stable), and sleeping better. And that's just the beginning. The benefits are, quite literally, endless.

It's not surprising, then, that one of the main benefits of strength training is a true expansion of one's range of motion; people who are strong move out into the world more freely and more adventurously, and they tend to see the possibilities instead of the pitfalls.

The benefits of strength-building for your muscles, joints, and ligaments may seem obvious, but it's worth reminding ourselves:

○ When you build muscle strength, your tendons and ligaments get stronger, too. This reduces your risk of injury.

○ Strength training builds muscle, increasing the amount of metabolically active tissue so your body burns more fat and becomes leaner.

○ When your muscles are strong, they are more responsive, so you are more agile.

If I sound like a real zealot for strength building, that's because I am. Resistance training is one of the best activities to keep you prime for life. It's the foundation of being fit. Or, more accurately, FITT.

FITT—THE FOUR-PART FORMULA FOR BUILDING STRENGTH

Before I walk you through the FITT program (which stands for frequency, intensity, time, and type) and specific strength-building exercises, I'd like to remind you, if you have any physical concerns or health problems, to please talk to your doctor or a physical therapist before you begin a strength-building program.

Here are the components of this program:

F = FREQUENCY of workouts. In order to get the maximum benefit of strength training, it's important to do it on a regular basis. Three nonconsecutive days a week is ideal, but 2 days a week will do the trick (once a week simply isn't enough). Your body responds best to resistance work when you give it a day to rest between workouts.

I = INTENSITY. Intensity is the level of exertion you bring to the exercise plan. This is usually calibrated by the number of repetitions of a particular exercise you're asked to complete. The goal, with any set, is to be in a state of fatigue that is called "near failure" when you complete the last rep. What that means is that your last rep should be the last one you know you can complete successfully (8 to 15 are the number of repetitions recommended by the American College of Sports Medicine for those new to resistance training). Body builders like to go all the way to "failure," but this is the "sport" in it for these serious athletes. But my goal is to have you succeed, not fail. Your strength-training goal is to build muscle for optimal function, not for bulk.

T = TIME. You will keep track of the time needed for each repetition, the number of times each exercise is performed, and the number of repetitions. Each time you perform an exercise it is called a "set." If you lift a dumbbell 10 times, you have performed one set of 10 repetitions. I recommend you lift on a count of 2 seconds and slowly lower on a count of 4 seconds. Time is also the rest you take between sets. If you perform two sets, a 2- to 3-minute rest between the sets provides the recovery time needed so that you can work hard on the second set. When you graduate to more than one set, you will be alternating between exercises for different muscles so that each muscle gets enough recovery time between repetitions.

T = TYPE. This refers to the type of exercise you'll be doing. For strength development, you can use dumbbells, resistance tubes, weight-training machines, or your own body weight (calisthenics). In the Prime for Life workouts you will be using resistance tubes and calisthenics.

Now that you know what the four basic components of the FITT process are, we'll move into the four phases of its execution. In Phase 1, you will learn the movements and practice them. You will begin with one set of each exercise.

THE FOUR PHASES OF THE FITT PLAN

Phase 1: Mastering the Basics

During the first month of strength training, you will be training your brain to recognize new movements. The goal of this first phase is to learn to execute each exercise properly and safely, and at the end of the month, they should be pretty automatic for you. After 1 month of practice, you will gradually increase the load, which will build your strength over time.

You'll begin with very little resistance or, in some cases, none. The important part of this phase is to really learn these basic skills so that you'll avoid injury when you increase resistance later on.

Phase 1 will begin changing how you move in the world, and your awareness of your own body. It will also be the beginning of a stronger, more supple you.

Phase 2: Building Strength

This second phase of the FITT program lasts 3 months. During the first 6 to 8 weeks of the program, your muscles will be getting stronger due to learning and better control of the muscles. After about 8 weeks, you will develop more mass. (If muscles have atrophied because you've been sedentary, you can actually "turn back the clock," restoring the muscle mass that has been lost.) You should start seeing some real changes with this. You will perform one set of 8 to 15 repetitions per exercise, resting between each exercise for 1 to 2 minutes. When you can perform 15 repetitions in two consecutive workouts on an exercise perfectly, then you'll increase the resistance during the next workout. By gradually increasing the resistance, you will likely need to decrease the number of repetitions you do, but this is normal, and the trade-off (more resistance, less time) is quite beneficial.

Phase 3: Adaptation

This third phase will last for 3 months. At this point, you continue with one set of the same exercises with 8 to 15 repetitions, using the highest resistance you used during each exercise in the second phase. During this period, your body adapts to these new levels of resistance and they become your new "normal." During this phase you will not change the resistance. After the first month of this phase, you'll begin decreasing recovery time between sets and start "circuit" training, which means alternating quickly between cardiovascular exercises and resistance exercises. This "changes up" the program while increasing its benefits. In between each exercise, you can walk, run, ride a stationary bike, or aerobic dance for 1 to 2 minutes. You will find it to be fun. Focus on moving continuously and briskly between the exercises. Don't do anything that causes joint pain—anywhere in your body. Use the BPES at moderate intensity or move as quickly as you can while still able to talk in short sentences—no more than *slightly* "huffy puffy."

Phase 4: Optional Increase

This final phase of the program is when you really take it on and make it your own. This phase lasts for 3 months. You begin increasing the number of sets to two per exercise. You will add only one set of each exercise at a rate of only two new and additional sets per week. Week 1, you'll only do the first two exercises with two sets. Week 2, you'll add a second set to the third and fourth exercises, and week 3 you'll add a second set to the fifth and sixth exercises. But to save time and begin increasing bone density, you will only be doing 6 to 12 repetitions, which means the resistance will be a little heavier. Rest for 2 minutes between sets on each exercise or alternate between two exercises at a time so that as one muscle group recovers, you work another muscle group before going back to the first. This way you make faster time through the workout by continually moving. When you can perform two sets of 12 repetitions on an exercise for two consecutive workouts, you will increase resistance the next workout. This corresponds roughly to the *BEST* study on mineral density (see Chapter 5). The exercises for your "core" will still include only one set, but you may add a few more repetitions (up to 15 to 20 on each).

After this year of getting fit, I recommend continuing with alternating between Phase 4 and Phase 3, but learn some new exercises to add variety. Three-month cycles allow gradual improvement and prevent burnout and injury. At this point (if your physician has deemed you able), in Phase 3 you can work at heavy intensity. Move as fast as you can sustain, at the "huffy-puffy" level of breathing.

THE FITT EXERCISES

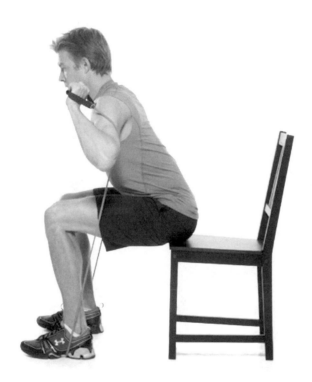

1. POTTY SQUAT

This is the single most important exercise for maintaining functional independence, and it is used by physical therapists when rehabilitating most knee injuries. Performed correctly, it is safe and works the muscles of the buttocks, quadriceps, hamstrings, erector spinae, shoulders, chest, and arms. Initially, you will practice it without any resistance other than your body weight. You should be wearing a good supportive running or walking shoe with the laces comfortably snug.

Before you start, imagine that you're hovering over a porta-potty. The goal is to move your derriere back—not down. This engages your powerful buttock muscles.

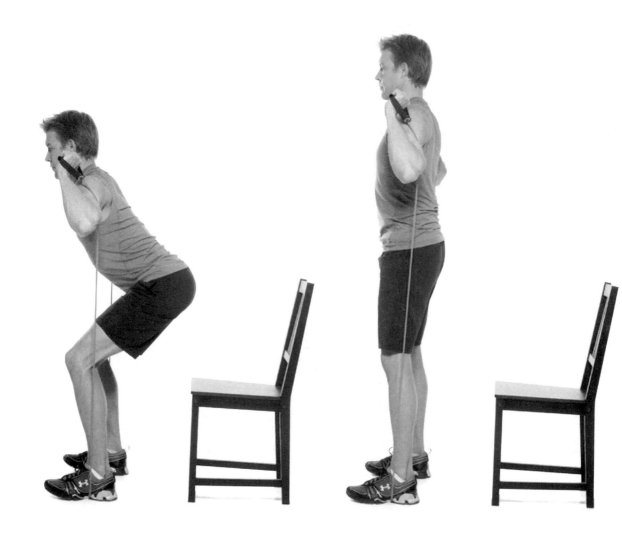

Start by standing in front of a chair as if you were about to sit down. March a few steps in place. Stop. Look down at your feet. Note the angle of the turnout of your feet. Now, sit down on the edge of the chair. Place your feet so that the outsides of your shoes are the same width apart as your hips. Adjust your feet so that the angle of turnout is about where it was when you stopped marching (symmetrical).

To rise, stiffen your abdomen and waist and keep your back completely straight. Reach forward for balance, getting your nose over your toes, and stand up by pushing down through your heels. Imagine a string pulling your chest up.

If possible, have a friend hold a yardstick against your spine to verify that you are keeping it straight. Stand up. Did your spine round? Keep practicing until you can do this with a straight spine.

Every time you do these squats, imagine a line that runs from the middle of your thighs to your knees. Site down from above, making sure the line ends *exactly* in the middle of your shoelaces for each knee. This is extremely important. If it's not in line, adjust your feet so that the thigh line is lined up exactly with your shoelaces. Knee pain in squats is almost invariably due to twisting (even slightly) in the knee. A slight deviation from this alignment usually makes the difference between pain and no pain. Also make sure your heels are directly below each knee at the base of the movement.

The Four Rules of Spine and Knee Protection for the Potty Squat Are:

1. Always keep your thigh EXACTLY in line with your shoelaces.
2. NEVER allow your knees to move directly over the end of your toes.
3. ALWAYS keep your spine straight; never round or flex it during lifting.
4. NEVER tolerate any pain or discomfort in your knees.

When you are able to perform this exercise consistently without pain, with your knees and your back in alignment, for at least 8 reps, try it without your arms extended in front of you. Instead, let your arms relax at your sides. To prevent yourself from falling back, you'll need to lean forward more. You should experience this exercise as one fluid movement of your hips and knees moving in concert.

If you can't master this exercise without knee pain, try using a higher chair. This limits the challenge to your quadriceps and makes good alignment easier for weaker thighs. Then when you can perform 15 repetitions without pain, use a slightly lower chair. The goal is to eventually and painlessly be able to rise from a low, soft chair beginning with your knees at about a right angle. If you just cannot perform this exercise without pain, see a physical therapist.

When you've mastered this without using your arms, you can add resistance tubing to the exercise. Stand with the middle of the tube under your arches. With an underhand grip, bend your elbows, pulling the handles in toward your shoulders. Swing your elbows up and in between the bands—push your elbows back. Relax your elbows down.

SOMETHING EXTRA WITH RESISTANCE TUBES

In some of the exercises that follow, I recommend using resistance tubes. These tubes are made by a number of companies. Some of the best are:

Spri Products (www.spriproducts.com) Xertubes and Xerings; 800-222-7774

Power Systems (www.power-systems.com) Versa-Tubes and Versa-O; 800-321-6975

The tubes come in various thicknesses. The thicker the band, the greater the resistance—each designated with a different color. They have handles on the ends for a comfortable grip. When you master 15 repetitions with a particular color, you graduate to the next, thicker tube of a different color. You can even double them up for even more resistance.

The bands weigh only a few ounces and are excellent for staying in shape when traveling. The colors, from easier to harder, are: yellow, green, red, blue, and black (or purple). Make sure you purchase an "anchor strap," a piece of nylon webbing that attaches to a door for "anchoring" the tube. Some individuals may eventually need to use two bands at a time (e.g., when you can do all the repetitions with purple, add a yellow one, too, then a green one with the purple, etc.).

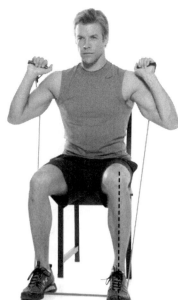

Always make certain that the midline of your thigh and center of your kneecap remain *exactly* in line with the midline of your shoes— no slight twisting!

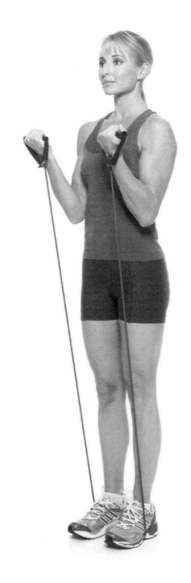

2. BICEPS CURLS

Stand on the tube with both feet. Keep your elbows against your waist with your arms straight and down at your sides. Exhale while curling your hands up toward your shoulders. Keep your wrists straight. Pause. Inhale, and slowly straighten your arms. (Don't allow your elbows to hyperextend.) Think of straightening your elbows, but not locking them.

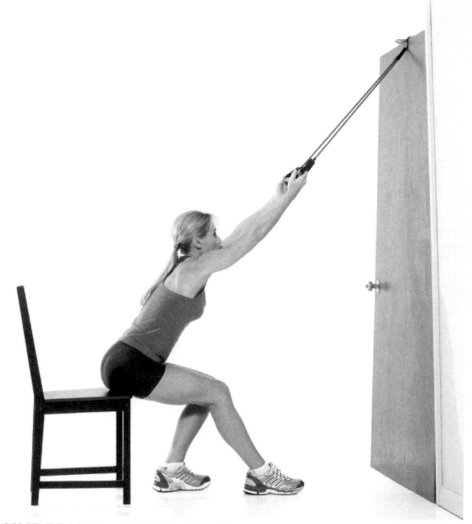

3. UNDERHAND PULLDOWN

For this exercise, you'll need a resistance tube and an anchor strap (a strap with a loop near the end and a "stop" on the end). Position the "stop" of the anchor handle up high behind an open door. Place the anchor strap close to the hinge side for safety. Close the door and tug on the anchor strap to make sure it won't move.

Now thread your tubing through the loop near the top of the anchor strap. Hold the handles on your tubing and step back with your arms straight until you place some tension on the tube. Have a chair behind you upon which to sit down. Lean forward on the chair with your arms extended up in line with the tube. Brace yourself with one foot in front, one in back. Hold the handles with a palms-up grip. Exhale, pulling down. Bring your hands to your chest, maintaining the palms-up grip. Pause. Then inhale, slowly resisting the tube back up to its starting position. It

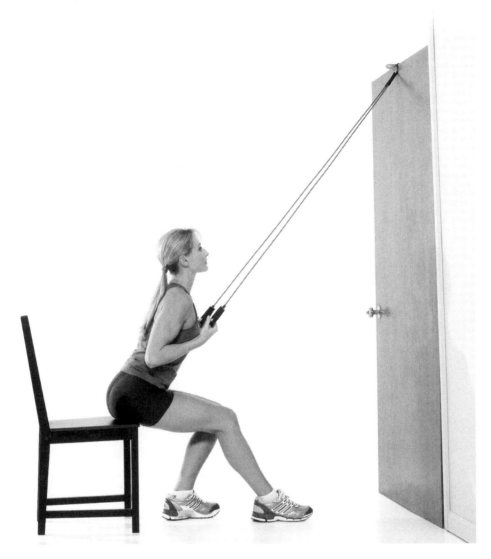

is important to allow your shoulder blades to rise up (upward rotation) toward your neck, but stay in control, resisting it all the way.

Focus on keeping the rest of the body stable—not moving. Keep the spine in line with the tube.

This exercise works the latissimus dorsi, teres major, and biceps and also stretches the downward rotators of the shoulder blades on the upstroke. These muscles are in the back and shoulders and are powerful muscles that help you swim, paddle a canoe, etc. This exercise is excellent for preventing rotator cuff injuries.

During the upstroke, let the tube stretch your shoulders up and out from your spine. (And remember, pain is a signal to stop!)

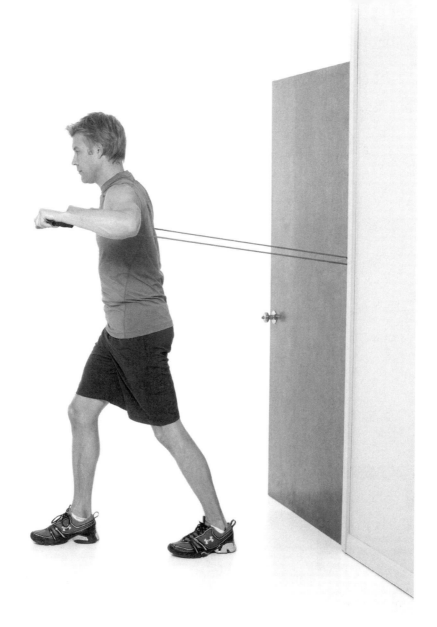

4. CHEST PRESS

Start with the lightest tube. Move the anchor strap down the hinge side of the door (it is less likely to come out than if it's on the doorknob side) to chest height. Face away from the door, with one foot in front for stability, putting tension on the tube. Hook the handles of the tubing with your thumbs, press the handles against your palms, and let the straps go under your arms.

Now, step out to put tension on the strap. Begin with your elbows at right angles. Your palms should be facing the floor and your forearms parallel to each

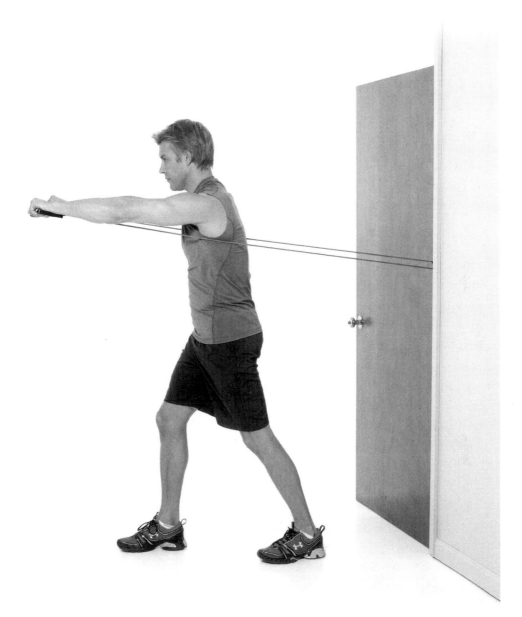

other. Do *not* let your elbows come back behind your waist—this can press the head of your humerus against the front of your shoulder capsule and biceps tendon, leading to a shoulder problem. Always place one foot in front of you and lean on that foot for safety.

Exhale as you push out, straightening your arms until your hands touch. Pause, then inhale SLOWLY, returning back to the starting position with your arms until, again, they are at a right angle out beside your chest and your forearms are parallel to each other and the floor. Pause, and then repeat. Perform 8 to 15 repetitions.

5. LATERAL SHOULDER RAISE IN EXTERNAL ROTATION IN THE PLANE OF THE SCAPULAE

We begin with this exercise to strengthen the supraspinatus muscle, the most commonly injured rotator cuff. That muscle is about the thickness of your little finger. To exercise it, you need very light resistance.

Practice the movement by standing with your back against a wall. Using NO resistance tube, slowly swing your hands up, with your thumbs up, about 30 to 40 degrees out from the wall. Stop when your arms are at shoulder height. Pause. Slowly lower your hands back down to your side. Repeat 8 to 15 times, trying for 15.

If that was easy and painless, the next time use the lightest resistance band (yellow). Start again, exhaling on the upstroke, and inhaling on the downstroke. Repeat. Perform 8 to 15 repetitions of this exercise. As with all the strength exercises, STOP before reaching failure or pain.

You should only begin increasing the resistance tubing when you can perform 15 repetitions. It doesn't matter if it takes several months. When you step up the resistance, you will need to be able to complete 8 to 15 repetitions.

Initially, this exercise will improve the function of your supraspinatus muscle, optimizing shoulder function. It trains you to work in the plane of the scapulae, the 30 to 40 degrees forward of the wall angle that is easier on the shoulders. The supraspinatus, as the most commonly injured rotator cuff, is progressively strengthened, and as resistance increases, the larger, overlying deltoid muscles are, too. You will develop strong shoulders that are less prone to injury.

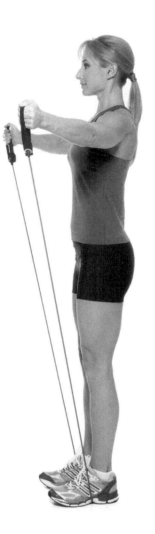

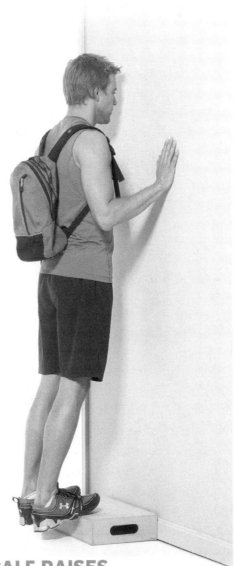

6. ECCENTRIC CALF RAISES

Stand on the edge of a step. Steady yourself for balance and safety. Exhale while lifting your heels to bring your full weight up onto your toes as high as you can while you count off 2 seconds ("one thousand one, one thousand two"). Inhale slowly, lowering your heels until you feel a stretch while you count off 6 seconds. Start with 8 repetitions and gradually build up to 15. When you can perform 15 reps without difficulty, begin lifting on both legs and then lowering on one leg. Do this for each leg. Again, start with 8 repetitions and gradually build up to 15. When this is easy, lift and lower on one leg or add a knapsack holding a 5-pound weight. Refer to page 117.

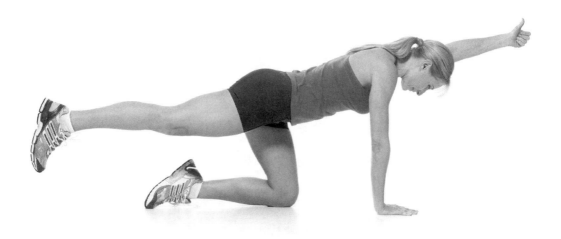

7. BIRD DOG

Level 1

This is an abdominal exercise as much as a spine strengthener. The belly and waist muscles—abdominus rectus, internal and external obliques, and transversus abdominus—are used to prevent movement of your spine. They are stabilizers more than movers.

On hands and knees, keep your spine as straight and flat as you can. Stiffen or brace your entire midsection. When braced and ready, slowly raise and extend your right leg straight back. Think of reaching back with your leg until it is in line with your spine, rather than lifting it. As you do so, exhale. Avoid arching or twisting your lower back. Pause for 5 to 8 seconds, continuing to avoid any arching or twisting. Don't hold your breath! You must develop the ability to use your core while breathing normally. Carefully lower your leg without moving your back. With practice you'll be rock solid and breathing comfortably. Repeat on the other side. Build up to 10 per side.

Now, perform the same movement, bracing your midsection as before. This time, extend the opposite arm in front of you. Again, do not allow your lower back to twist or arch. (You may need to have a friend tell you if you are in alignment or do this next to a mirror.) Do 8 to 15 repetitions on each side. This is an excellent lower back stabilization exercise.

Level 2

In the advanced bird dog, extend your left leg and your right arm straight out. Keep your lower back straight by bracing your midsection. There must be no twisting or arching. Repeat on the opposite side. Over time, build up to 15 reps per side, holding each repetition for 5 seconds, while remaining aware of your breathing. Unlike most strength exercises, do not exhale up and inhale down. Rather, exhale up and breathe softly and naturally as you hold the position. Do not arch or twist your lower back. Rather than reaching up with your hand and foot, think of elongating without any movement of your pelvis or trunk or lower back.

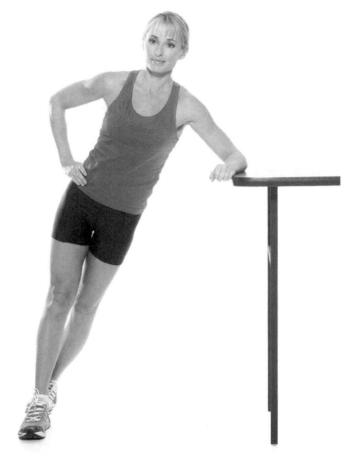

8. SIDE PLANK

Level 1: Against a Countertop

With this exercise, it's very important to wear supportive shoes with a good grip so you don't slip!

Lean against a kitchen countertop on your elbow. Place one foot in front of the other. Keep your body in an absolute straight line and hold your weight evenly distributed between both feet. As in all core exercises, brace your midsection first, but try to breathe naturally. Hold the position for 5 to 8 seconds.

Now face the other direction and repeat.

Do this 10 times on each side.

Never get too close to failure on this one. You are training your waist muscles (external obliques, internal obliques, transversus abdominus, and quadratus lumborum) to stabilize your lumbar spine, protecting it from injury.

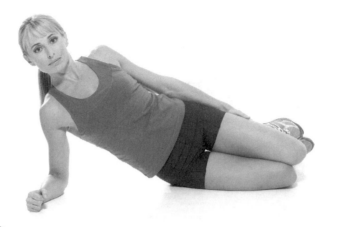

Level 2

At a lower angle, or when your body is more horizontal, this exercise is more challenging. Again, brace, breathe, and avoid going to failure. Start on the floor with your hips bent and knees a bit forward and spine straight—no lazy slumping spine. As your hips come off the floor, press them forward so that when you're up your spine is straight and in line with your thighs. Build up to at least 5 seconds with 8 to 15 reps per side.

If this bothers your shoulder, here is an alternative exercise.

Rest your head on a pillow. Lie on your side and lift both legs up an inch. Hold for 5 to 8 seconds. Build gradually to at least 8 to 15 reps per side. Breathe naturally as you hold the position!

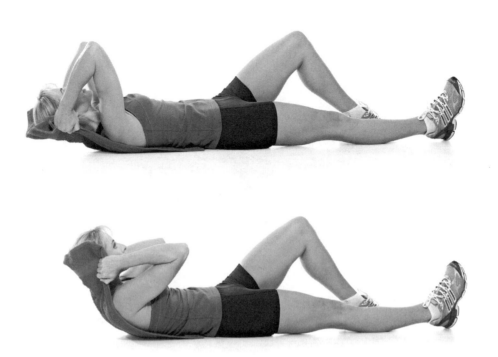

9. CURLUP

Lie down on a soft, carpeted floor. Put a hand towel under you. Lie on the towel—it should extend from under your back to the top of your head. Bend one knee up and extend your other leg out on the floor. This relaxes your hip flexors. Hold the towel beside your ears tightly to support your head.

This is a "mini curlup," not a full one. (The full one can place excessive force on your lumbar spine and shorten your abdominals.) The towel is used to support your head and prevent you from bending your neck forward. Your neck should remain straight and in line with your upper back. Your lower back should remain in a normal, slight curve.

Brace or stiffen your midsection and do NOT distend your belly. Lift your head slightly by holding the corners of the towel. Rock gently up onto your upper back. Do not press your lower back down or tilt or move your pelvis. Your head "rides up," supported by the towel, saving the neck from strain. Hold for 5 to 10 seconds and breathe softly and naturally in and out.

Build up gradually until you can hold each repetition for 5 to 8 seconds and repeat up to 15 times. You should not have to reverse your leg position if the legs are truly relaxed, but you can, if you choose.

Alternative Abdominal Exercise or If You Have Osteoporosis

If there is osteoporosis in the lumbar spine, curling up compresses the spinal bodies together where most bone weakness tends to occur. For that reason, no doctor or physical therapist would recommend that you do curlups if you have spinal osteoporosis. Lie on your back with your knees bent and your feet flat on the floor. Stiffen your abdomen and waist. Do *not* distend your belly. Exhale as you lift your left knee until it is directly over your left hip. Avoid pushing down with the other leg. Pause. Keep it there. Now also lift your right knee up over the right hip. Focus on keeping your lower back exactly the same—no arch or pelvic tilt. Your breathing should be natural and soft.

Slowly lower your left leg back down. Slowly lower your right leg back down.

Repeat, lifting with the right first. Alternate sides, and gradually build up to 10 to 15 reps per leg.

As in all core-stabilizing exercises, never go to failure or fatigue. This exercise does tend to use the hip-flexing muscles that attach to the front of the lumbar spine, so if you encounter any lower back pain, discontinue.

WASHBOARD ABS?

I know a lot of people—men, especially—think that abdominal curls are necessary if they want to build up their abdominal "washboard muscle," the abdominus rectus. This is just one long muscle that connects the bottom of the breastbone to the pubic bone. (Contrary to what some people believe, there is no such thing as an "upper abdominal" and a "lower abdominal.")

It's true that the curlup is a good way to build this muscle, but I wouldn't recommend it for anyone who has osteoporosis. The alternative abdominal exercise also exercises the abdominus rectus, but without curling the trunk at all. So you get the benefit of working out those abdominal muscles, but without the threat of injury to the spine.

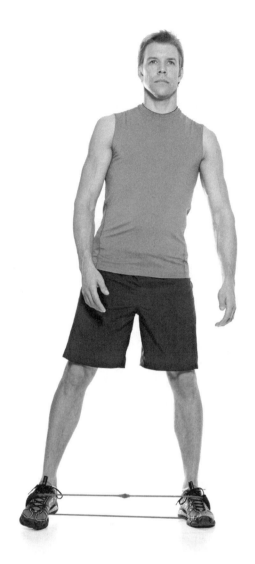

10. GLUTEUS MEDIUS STRENGTHENER

The hip abductor muscle, the gluteus medius, is a muscle on the side of the hip that functions to swing your leg out away from the midline. You have a pair of these muscles (one for each hip), and they are important for preventing hip adduction. (Hip adduction is when the thigh and knee come into the midline of the body and cause excessive twisting in the knee and the lower back.) The hip abductor muscle also needs to be strong to maintain optimal alignment of the hip.

You will need a resistance tubing ring for this exercise (or you can make a knot in a piece of straight tubing to form a ring). Start with the lightest resistance if you have a history of knee problems; otherwise, you can move directly to the ring with the second level of resistance.

Place the ring around your feet. To provide greatest resistance, the ring should be under your arches with the black reinforcement tubes around the sides of your shoes. (Don't put the ring around your ankles; you could injure yourself if you lose your balance.)

Step slowly to the left, but no more than 18 inches or the band may break. Now, slowly bring your right leg in, resisting the pull of the tube. As you step to the left with your left leg, your right leg follows after. Continue moving for 8 to 12 steps to the left. Now take the same number of steps back to the right, returning to your starting place.

Now repeat. Go to the left for 8 to 12 steps, then return to the starting point at your right. Maintain a tall, upright posture, with your knees only very slightly bent. Keep your spine straight.

If you can't avoid bending your lower back to the side, you need to use a lower resistance tube. Over time, build up to two sets of 8 to 15 repetitions, alternating with a different exercise between sets.

A SMOOTH LAUNCH

I want to end this chapter by congratulating you for your determination to get stronger—it's the best thing you can do to keep yourself fit and active. But it sometimes comes with a cost.

Anytime we start a new fitness program, we're bound to experience some soreness, and it's important to point out that this is normal—it is not a sign of injury at all! When we work our muscles in new ways, we "stress" them and there is inevitably going to be a bit of sensation around this. (This is a big reason why alternating days is so crucial to your strength-building program—it allows your muscles time to regroup.)

One of the pitfalls of strength training is that after a day or two, your muscles feel sore. It's called delayed onset muscle soreness, or DOMS. Lifting a dumbbell up to your shoulder by bending your elbow in a biceps curl uses your biceps brachii muscle. That muscle shortens. As you lower your muscle, and your elbow straightens again, your muscle lengthens. It is the eccentric phase of a muscle contraction—or the "un-contraction" of the motion—that causes DOMS. As a result, you may feel quite sore for several days. DOMS is a very mild form of muscle strain.

Anytime a muscle is strained, it goes through the process of inflammation. This means pain, stiffness, and swelling. In mild soreness, it is okay to continue your 3-day-a-week program, but do not attempt to increase the resistance for several weeks after this. In a severe strain from injury, you need to allow the tissues to rest and avoid all painful movements. So with your resistance program, if using the same or slightly lighter resistance doesn't hurt, go ahead and stick to your schedule. Avoid pain. This is part of the reason why your strength-training program should alternate between days of rest and activity. After the rest period, moving around usually makes you feel better. If you can move without pain, do it. It gets that healing blood flowing to your injured area. Also, you're a lot less likely to feel soreness in that muscle again as long as you continue exercising it.

The soreness is harmless. In fact, think of it as an indication of progress. As the muscle goes through a regenerative process, it is laying down new protein and preparing to be stronger. So . . . keep exercising. Just don't increase resistance right away. (Research has shown that you are likely to be a bit weaker for up to 2 weeks after DOMS begins.)

By the way, I don't recommend taking nonsteroidal anti-inflammatories such as aspirin or ibuprofen for relief of soreness. In decreasing inflammation (and yes, pain) they decrease muscle healing from DOMS. Instead, try putting some ice on the sore area for 15 minutes (no more, as you can literally cause frostbite and tissue damage). Ice is a wonderful anesthetic agent. You can also take Tylenol (acetaminophen) in small doses, as it quells pain without affecting inflammation.

I haven't found any surefire, magic treatments for sore muscles other than one—the magic of time. Be patient. Smart, fit people learn to incorporate other types of exercise into their lives when they're a bit sore. There is always some type of painless exercise to keep you fit while you're healing (such as walking or gently swimming).

Any soreness you may experience will fade quickly as you deepen your program and the days and repetitions begin to add up. Before you know it, you'll feel fantastic and you'll never want to miss a day of strength training again!

CHAPTER FIVE

STRONG BONES

"Most people don't realize that
osteoporosis and thinning bones are
preventable. And, the good news is that no
matter what the condition of your bones,
there are things you can do to make them
stronger and help reverse the condition."
—*Miriam Nelson*, **Strong Women, Strong Bones**

Your skeleton is truly a marvel of architecture and engineering. Made up of 206 bones, the adult skeleton supports your body and allows you to move. It also provides protection for our organs and soft tissues. Without a skeleton, we'd be like giant jellyfish washed to shore—wobbly sacks of flesh, filled with fluid and organs. Instead, we have an amazing framework of bones, which provides the scaffolding upon which our muscles and organs connect.

Our skeletal system is made up of bone (hard tissue) and cartilage (soft tissue) that work in concert, allowing us to move smoothly and fluidly, rather than jangle along, like a rickety tangle of sticks. The calcified (hard) bones in our skeleton also work with our circulatory system; both red and white blood cells are created inside bone. The muscles that attach to bones, when activated, contract and allow us to move. It's an amazing system that most of us take for granted—until we experience some difficulty in moving.

YOUR EVER-CHANGING FRAME

There are many ways the skeletal system protects your internal organs from injury. Your rib cage cradles your heart and lungs, shielding them from harm. Your skull protects your brain. Bones provide the support and leverage to walk, swim, and play. Bones are also a reserve for calcium, the vital mineral used in muscle contractions and other metabolic processes.

Bone is living, dynamic tissue that is constantly undergoing change. In fact, it is constantly breaking itself down and rebuilding in a process known as remodeling—that is, the body actually discards old bone and builds new bone. This process continues throughout our lifetime.

Two kinds of bone cells, osteoclasts and osteoblasts, perform opposite tasks in remodeling. Osteoclasts release substances that break down the structural part of bone, which releases calcium into the bloodstream when it is needed. This phase of remodeling, called resorption, lasts about 2 to 3 weeks. Osteoblasts synthesize new bone in a slower process with a span of about 2 to 3 months.

Remodeling enables bone to heal to 100 percent of its original strength in a normal, healthy person. It allows calcium to be released into the bloodstream or stored again in the bones. In younger people, osteoblasts tend to be more active than osteoclasts, so during our formative years our bones increase in size and strength. (Children are born with almost 300 bones. Many of them fuse together as we mature, becoming stronger and denser.) As we age, the process tends to reverse. In most people, bone density and strength gradually diminish. Osteoporosis occurs when degradation occurs faster than rebuilding.

In our late thirties our bones are at their strongest. After that, they begin losing minerals and density at a slow, steady rate, becoming more porous and brittle over time. Our sex hormones, estrogen and testosterone, are also important in maintaining bone strength. During menopause, with a sudden drop in estrogen levels, women begin losing bone at a faster rate than they did the decade before. When men suffer a decline in testosterone, they, too, experience a decline in bone density.

One of the remarkable things about bone is its ability to adapt to stress. When pressure (stress) is applied, your bone forms supporting strands of connective tissue called trabeculae, which provide the bone with the additional support it needs to bear the load. Here's how it works: Every time you take a step, you apply stress to your skeleton that radiates up through your feet, legs, and hips, through the pelvis, and on up your spine. Simply walking puts this kind of stress on your skeleton, and that's a good thing. (When you walk, you are putting pressure equivalent to 1 to 1½ times your own body weight on your skeleton. When you run, you up that pressure to 2 to 6 times your body weight!) The more of this healthy, weight-bearing pressure you apply, the more beautiful, lacy trabeculae your skeleton builds to support your work. (Paleontologists are even able to determine the muscularity of a Neanderthal body based on an examination of the muscle-attachment points on the skeleton.)

OSTEOPOROSIS: THE SCOURGE OF THE SKELETON

We all know that osteoporosis is one of the most dreaded diseases of old age. It is also one of the most common. In this country alone, more than 10 million people over the age of 50 have osteoporosis, and more than 34 million people have the precursor condition, osteopenia. These numbers are daunting for many reasons, not the least of which is that they may lead people to believe that developing osteoporosis is inevitable.

The World Health Organization defines osteoporosis as "bone mineral density 2½ standard deviations below that of a young person of the same gender." Osteopenia, the early stages of osteoporosis, is a "low bone density between 1 and 2½ standard deviations below the mean of a young person."

Here's the good news: Osteoporosis is not only preventable, but it is also controllable and even, to a degree, reversible. The first line of defense is to determine whether you are at risk for developing this debilitating disease—or whether you already have it.

The greatest threat posed by osteoporosis is the risk of falling and fracturing a bone. There's even the risk of suffering a spontaneous fracture! (This can happen with someone with severely fragile and weakened bones that have lost their capacity for weight bearing.) The most common fractures associated with osteoporosis occur in the hip, the back (spine), and the wrist. Fully one out of two women will

WHAT PUTS US AT RISK FOR DEVELOPING OSTEOPOROSIS?

Age: Yes, age is a significant factor—but not because we're chronologically older. It's because, as we age, we tend to engage in fewer weight-bearing and strength-building activities. So the increase in risk of osteoporosis is partly attributable to our lifestyle choices!

Decreasing hormone levels: This applies to both men and women. Hormones help our bones absorb vital nutrients, such as calcium and vitamin D. As we age, and our hormone levels decrease, so does the nutrient load of our bones.

Being sedentary: When you're inactive, you deprive your skeleton of the stress that it needs to remain healthy and robust. A lifestyle that doesn't include strength-training and weight-bearing activities will put you at greater risk for osteoporosis when you become older.

Smoking: Studies have shown that smoking reduces the blood supply to bones and that nicotine slows the production of bone-forming cells (osteoblasts) and impairs the absorption of calcium. With less bone mineral, smokers develop osteoporosis. Women who take estrogen replacement therapy—which generally helps maintain or improve bone mass—won't get the same benefits if they're smokers. It's been shown that smoking actually reduces the protective effect of estrogen replacement therapy.

suffer a fracture like this at some point during her life. Men will, too, though the statistics are lower. According to some studies, as many as one-quarter to one-fifth of men are at risk. In the United States, more than 1.5 million fractures a year are attributed to osteoporosis. One-quarter of those are hip fractures.

When I worked in a hospital, I met many women who had suffered hip fractures due to osteoporosis. Those who were treated with surgery or a hip replacement tended to recover well. But there were others with complicated fractures who were never able to get back to the level of bone strength they had before the fracture. It was difficult to watch these women, so active and vital one day, become seriously incapacitated the next. I can't even imagine what this must have been like for them.

Fractures in the elderly bring on a host of other complications that can include

Drinking soda, caffeine, or alcohol in excess: Researchers aren't quite sure why drinking these beverages in excess increases your risk for developing osteoporosis, but evidence suggests that they limit the ability of nutrients to be absorbed by bone. For example, soda contains phosphoric acid, which can cause the leeching of calcium from bones.

Low levels of calcium and vitamin D: A diet low in these nutrients weakens bones. Vitamin D deficiency is a leading cause of osteoporosis, even for women taking calcium supplements. This is because vitamin D is needed to facilitate the absorption of calcium. We can get vitamin D with just 15 minutes a day of sunlight, but most of us aren't doing that. Individuals who use sunblock should be especially careful to get enough vitamin D in their diet or through supplements. Many women should be checked for vitamin D deficiency and take a supplement accordingly.

Taking certain medications: Some medications, such as corticosteroids—when taken over a long period of time—increase the risk of developing osteoporosis.

Body frame size: A small, light skeleton is at greater risk for bone density loss. That's because there is less natural weight bearing on that frame.

blood clotting or bone chip dislodgement, both of which can lead to stroke; septicemia (a serious blood infection); pneumonia (a side effect of being immobile); and even death (24 percent of hip-fracture patients die within 1 year). For reasons not understood, men have a higher mortality rate from hip fractures than women do.

Osteoporosis can also put you at risk for vertebral fractures. When you see a woman hunched over with a hump in her upper spine, a "dowager's hump," that woman is actually suffering from a broken back! Unlike a wrist, hip, or other joint, a broken back is very tough to treat; the only option is immobilization, and this is very difficult to achieve. Vertebral fractures are also excruciatingly painful.

On top of all that, the 6 or so weeks of bed rest following a serious fracture cause serious "deconditioning" in older patients, which includes an accelerated loss of bone density.

When and How to Be Screened for Osteoporosis

The U.S. Preventive Services Task Force recommends osteoporosis screening for all women over the age of 65. But, because bone density diminishes so dramatically during menopause, Canyon Ranch recommends that all women be screened, even those who have not yet reached menopause. Getting an early baseline measurement will help you get a sense of where you are on the bone density continuum. For women, this is especially important because a premenopause screening gives a baseline value that can be compared with postmenopausal bone density values. If there's loss of bone density, it will be readily apparent in the before–after comparison. Early detection leads to early treatment and the best possible outcome.

Measuring Bone Density

The gold standard for measuring bone mineral density (BMD) is the use of an extraordinary piece of technology called Dual Energy X-ray Absorptiometry (DEXA). Although it utilizes x-rays, the radiation exposure is less than you'd get flying across the country. A DEXA scan provides detailed information about the state of bone density in the total body or in specific problem areas, such as the hip or lumbar spine.

Knowing your bone density level allows your physician to accurately assess your risk of fractures. For example, someone in the beginning stages of osteopenia in the low back has a 2.3 times greater likelihood of breaking her hip than someone with normal bone density in that area. If there's osteopenia in the hip, risk for fracture is 2.6 times higher than normal. If you have osteoporosis, your risk of a spinal fracture is 8 times higher than normal, and the risk of hip fracture is 11 times greater. As these statistics clearly show, having strong bones is more important than most of us can fathom.

Strong Bones Keep Osteoporosis at Bay

Before you embark on your bone-building weight-training program, here are a few important things to bear in mind:

○ If you use weight-training machines at the gym or at home, they should be the kinds that support your spine. These include those that support your *entire* spine, such as the equipment used for leg presses, chest presses, overhead presses, etc. Gym attendants may not have

WHAT DOES THE DEXA DO?

Dual Energy X-ray Absorptiometry (DEXA) is a noninvasive, painless way to get a measurement of how many minerals are in a specific bone site. This test is crucial to detecting the onset of osteoporosis in those who are symptom free. From an interpretation of the scan results, a physician can:

- Detect low bone density before a person breaks a bone.

- Predict a person's chances of fracture in the future.

- Confirm a diagnosis of osteoporosis when a person already has a broken bone.

- Determine whether a person's bone density is decreasing, increasing, or staying the same.

- Help monitor a person's response to treatment.

Who Should Take the DEXA?

- Premenopausal women (to establish a baseline value to compare with postmenopausal BMD).

- A postmenopausal woman under age 75 with one or more risk factors for osteoporosis.

- A man age 50 to 70 with one or more risk factors for osteoporosis.

- Any woman over age 65, without any known risk factor.

- A man over age 70, without any known risk factor.

- A woman or man over 50 who has broken a bone.

- A woman going through menopause with certain risk factors.

- A postmenopausal woman who has stopped hormone therapy.

Based on the determination of bone mineral density (BMD) from the DEXA assessment, your doctor will let you know your risk factors for osteopenia and osteoporosis.

THE *BEST* STUDY OF BONE DENSITY

The BEST study (which stands for Bone Estrogen Strength Training study) was conducted in Arizona between 1995 and 2001 and is considered to be a seminal study in osteoporosis. The study looked at 266 sedentary postmenopausal women, ages 44 to 66, all in relatively good health. The subjects were all nonsmokers. About half of them were on hormone replacement therapy; the others were not. Every participant took a daily calcium supplement. The subjects' bone density was measured prior to the test using the Bone Mineral Density (BMD) test.

Participants in the BEST study were divided into two groups, half taking hormone replacement therapy and half not. The object of the study was to determine what effect weight-bearing exercise had on bone mineral density (BMD) when the only variable was exercise. So one group on each team (those taking hormones, and those not) undertook a strength-training program, while the others had no regular strength training at all. Exercisers performed supervised aerobic, weight-bearing, and weight-lifting exercises, three times per week in community-based exercise facilities. To encourage and maintain interest in exercise for one year, the women in the strength-training group participated in social support programs resulting in a high level of adherence.

The findings were startling. The participants in both groups who *exercised*— whether they were taking hormones or not—had markedly improved bone density in their hips and low backs, the areas of focus for the study. (The hormone-taking group showed a slightly higher, but not significant, level of improvement.) Among the *nonexercisers,* the hormone-taking group showed a slight increase in bone density while the other group showed no improvement at all—or, even worse, showed a decrease in bone density.

The study powerfully showed that a dramatic increase in bone density and strength can occur with regular, weight-bearing exercise.

training in dealing with osteoporosis, but they will be able to show you the safe way to use these machines.

○ Strengthening the major muscles of your arms, shoulders, legs, hips, and back extensors helps your posture and keeps you from rounding over. A strong, straight musculoskeletal system helps maintain strong bones.

○ Avoid the lower back strengthening machines or lower back extension exercises in which you move from flexion of the spine to extension. Also avoid the abdominal and waist strength machines. When you do exercises on these machines, you put excessive force on your lumbar spine. That can be dangerous.

○ The seated leg press machine, in which you sit with your entire spine supported and push with your legs, is safe for your spine and strengthens your hips and thighs. Avoid moving the seat in too close; this can force your pelvis to tilt, thus flexing your spine.

○ Lower back exercises don't increase spinal bone density very well. Weight-bearing exercises, performed while standing, are better. If you fall into the category of osteopenia, the potty squat is ideal for improving the two areas with the most potential risk for fracture—your hips and spine. The resistance is carried straight down through your spine into the hips, which has been found to help BMD the most. This is an example of "axial loading," in which the resistance is carried through the length of a bone or the spine.

○ For people with healthy bones, a rounded over (kyphotic) spine is often caused by short abdominal muscles. The modified abdominal curl is not recommended for individuals with osteoporosis in the spine, but the alternative abdominal exercise in Chapter 4 is an excellent way to work these muscles safely.

○ Never use abdominal exercises on gym balls if you believe you have osteoporosis. A fall from the ball could be devastating.

○ Learning to "log roll" is essential when you're getting in and out of bed. It keeps you from placing excessive stress on your spine. When you roll over in bed or lie down, always focus on stiffening your trunk and rolling your whole body together like a log so that you don't twist your spine. For example, if you are lying on your back, bend your knees up. Reach across your body with your left hand. To turn onto your left side, reach and roll to your left side while simultaneously dropping both knees to the left.

Weight Training to Build Bone Density

People at lowest risk for developing osteoporosis are those who optimally stress their bones on a regular basis. Several studies have shown that athletes who participate in high-impact activities or lift heavy weights tend to have significantly greater bone density than the rest of us.

Jumping sports such as volleyball and gymnastics tend to promote good bone density. Olympic weight lifters, who perform sudden, rapid movements with heavy weights, are off the charts in bone density. Although none of us needs to strive for this kind of intensity in weight training, the example of these elite athletes teaches us that a strong body builds strong bones.

Nonetheless, we still have a lot to learn about the specific ways different exercises and activities affect bone density. But the word is out: Weight-bearing exercise is essential for maintaining and building strong bones. This includes walking, running, and jumping—in fact, any exercise that imparts gravitational force and some amount of axial (long bone) loading.

Unfortunately, walking alone may not give your bones all the strength building they need. One study of postmenopausal women found that the benefits of walking peaked after 6 weeks, yet it takes several years to significantly rebuild bone density. So other forms of exercise are necessary.

Running, for instance, is better for bone building because it can provide pressure of up to 5 or 6 times your body weight, particularly when you're running downhill. But for those of us over 50, running might not be the best choice because it can cause a lot of injuries. The good news is that there are safer and just as effective ways of getting your weight-bearing activity.

One of the interesting findings of the BEST study was that it showed heavy resistance with fewer repetitions was more effective than lighter resistance at more repetitions in building bone density and strength. Unlike prior studies that used more traditional recommendations of 8 to 12 or 10 to 15 repetitions, this study had the women perform 6 to 8 reps. When they could perform two sets of 8 repetitions on an exercise, the resistance was slightly increased the next workout.

Other studies have shown, too, that it takes more resistance and fewer repetitions to increase BMD. (In line with these results, in Phase 4 of the Prime for Life strength program, I recommend that you do 6 to 12 repetitions.) But the idea of adding weights to our workouts can be daunting—even frightening—for some of us. That's why I'm such a huge fan of resistance bands, which provide the weight load without the added risks associated with free weights or certain types of exercise equipment.

Nervous or not, it's important that we keep an open mind when it comes to weight training.

Jenny's STORY

Jenny was a 58-year-old woman who'd been coming to the Life Enhancement Program for a number of years. Five years before her latest visit, she had discovered that she had osteopenia—the early stages of osteoporosis. I love working with Jenny. She's enthusiastic and hardworking, and a great listener.

When Jenny got the diagnosis, she immediately gave up her diet soda habit. (It has been found that women who drink a lot of diet soda have a high risk of accelerated bone loss.) Jenny also upped her calcium intake and began weight training. In addition, she started taking a medication for bone health.

Initially, Jenny was hesitant to lift anything heavier than the 3-pound "beauty bells" she used at home. (This is an expression I use for any weight under 5 pounds; it's just not enough to have an impact on your program.) With encouragement, she gradually increased her weight load. Over 5 years, she progressed so much that she began to use, routinely, a resistance level of 45 pounds, either with gym equipment or with an equivalent resistance band.

At first, Jenny was afraid that she'd turn into a female Arnold Schwarzenegger, but today she looks quite attractive and lean. Most important, she tells me every chance she gets how great she feels and that the benefits of weight training have crept into every corner of her life.

"Everything is easier," she told me. "My endurance is better and I can lift my 2-year-old grandson up without a second thought."

Jenny's transformation didn't happen overnight, but it did happen. She's now off all medication for the osteopenia and will use strength training and nutrition to keep the osteoporosis at bay for as long as possible.

Where Weight Training Takes You

We know that a weight-training program must be of high intensity to promote bone regeneration, but as with anything else, we start reasonably and build up our weight load as we get stronger. Weight training does not need to be dangerous; in fact, it is quite safe if done properly. All you need is a month or so of practicing the exercises so that you learn to do them correctly and safely. After that, they'll be second nature and you'll do them spontaneously and with great focus.

During the initial phase of bone strengthening, you'll need to use lighter weights and higher repetitions to allow your muscles, ligaments, and tendons to get used to their new role. Once you become proficient at the first level, you will naturally progress to the next.

Strength Training and Osteoporosis

Although it's been shown by numerous studies that progressive resistance (strength) training can prevent and even reverse osteoporosis, the question is, how much do you need?

For measurable results, a minimum of 6 to 8 months of strength training is necessary. For *optimal* results, think of this as a 2-year project. If you have osteoporosis or osteopenia, it didn't happen overnight, but every workout makes you healthier and moves your bone density in the right direction.

No one is quite certain yet how intensively you should exercise once you are diagnosed with relatively advanced osteoporosis. Severe osteoporosis may create such fragile bones that they break with minimal movements. If your spine is weak, great force is placed on your vertebrae, compressing them, when you bend forward. This can, and does, cause compression fractures. (They're among the most painful fractures and they're difficult to treat.) It is imperative that you keep your spine straight. Yoga may be especially risky for you. Use meditation to achieve the same mental state, but skip the spinal contortions that may cause severe harm.

So, if you do have osteoporosis, it is essential that you ask your doctor and physical therapist for advice about strengthening exercise before you make it part of your life. It's also important to ask your doctor if medication could help you. These meds may include biphosphonates such as Fosamax, Boniva, Actonel, or Reclast. Hormone replacement therapy may also help, as well as calcium supplementation.

You can still do some resistance training if you have osteoporosis, but it's absolutely essential that you discuss this first with your physician and get his or her blessing. Unfortunately, we're not able to accurately predict the safe stress load that's needed to improve bones based on their deviation below normal. However, the American College of Sports Medicine does recommend gentle strength training for individuals with osteoporosis.

Please Remember . . .

○ If you have osteoporosis in your spine, never do situps, crunches, or any exercise that flexes you forward or twists your spinal column. This includes yoga, Pilates, Gyrotonics, tennis, and golf. Again, this diagnosis means that your vertebral bodies are so fragile that they are in danger of crumbling! Flexing or twisting the spine places maximum force on them.

○ If you are worried that you can't keep your tummy in shape, don't be. Crunches and situps generally train you to have poor posture anyway. The alternative abdominal exercise in Chapter 4 works better and won't harm your spine. Keep your back straight!

○ If you have a diagnosis of osteoporosis in your hips, it's important to understand how to target that region with weight training. Working muscles that are attached to your hip may help, but so will long-bone (axial) loading. A leg press machine applies axial loading through your femur into your hip, but the potty squat will load the hips and spine. A squat provides axial loading through the spine and hips, but you need to be extra careful to keep your knees safe and your spine in good alignment. Study the potty squat in Chapter 4 carefully (see page 63) and read Chapter 8.

○ You must discuss medications with your doctor. There has been enormous improvement in drugs that treat osteoporosis. For now, make sure you're taking enough calcium, keep exercising using appropriate and safe movements, avoid those colas, and be patient. Bones do get stronger.

What's Coming Down the Road

There are exciting and promising new lines of thinking regarding movement and treatment of osteoporosis. One that's very promising is the use of vibration to increase bone density. Many fitness "experts" are already recommending use of vibration devices with and without strength training. Research has determined that vibration does increase bone mineral density, and the optimum amounts necessary have been established. For now, more research needs to be done to determine whether vibration is okay for cartilage and your spine.

As I write, there are likely many new studies under way regarding how to use strength and weight training to combat osteoporosis. So stay tuned!

In the Meantime:

○ Wear shoes that give you good support and keep you close to the earth—avoid high heels.

○ Talk to your doctor about getting a baseline BMD screening.

○ Begin exercises that will promote your strength, flexibility, and overall level of fitness.

○ Avoid any activities that stress your bones, joints, or muscles in painful ways.

○ Avoid exercises that encourage you to bend forward—this means no more situps!

○ Avoid extreme twisting at the waist.

○ If you haven't stopped already, quit smoking.

○ Talk to your doctor about hormone replacement therapy or other medications that will promote bone health.

○ Make sure you have enough calcium and vitamin D in your diet so that your bones will be well nourished.

My goal is to help you feel the absolute best you can with the body you've got. I know that, regardless of your age, your current state of health, or your level of fitness, you can and will improve your bone health. All it takes is the desire, some effort, and a bit of patience. When your bones are strong, you will be prime for life.

CHAPTER SIX

YOUR FOOT AND ANKLE

"When our feet hurt, we hurt all over."
—*Socrates*

"The human foot is a masterpiece of
engineering and a work of art."
—*Leonardo da Vinci*

Your body's structure rests on a double foundation—your feet. Look at them and appreciate their extraordinary job. How many miles have they traveled? Look at their soles. The treads are as good as ever, though perhaps tough and calloused. And consider your ankles. How many times have they had to bend, swing, and swivel to help propel you along a track or assist you in keeping your balance? Feet are practical, hardworking, and longer lasting than any set of tires.

From ankles to toes, your feet have one function: Whether you're moving or standing, they provide a safe, stable base of support. They can negotiate all sorts of terrain. Uneven, slippery, sandy, or soft, your feet adapt. They also work in a way that allows the long bones in your leg to rotate in response to demands from the joints above—your knees and your hips.

We average more than 3 million steps per year. Talk about mind-boggling!

Your foot contains 26 bones, many articulations, tendons, and muscles. Six nerves wind their way through the ankle, heel, arch, and toes of each foot. (No wonder a foot massage feels so good!) Feet are your base for continued exercise and movement, and of course they carry a lot of responsibility for helping you maintain balance. (If the nerves in our feet are damaged, it compromises our ability to maintain our balance and stay upright.) In each part of the foot, and in many of the nerves, things can go wrong, causing you a great deal of discomfort.

Most of our foot problems peak between the ages of 40 and 60 and can be prevented. But for prevention to be effective, we must learn to appreciate our feet enough to get help as soon as we feel a change that slows us down or causes pain.

We can thank our feet by wearing shoes that fit well, using shoes that work best for specific activities, paying attention to early pain, and keeping our feet strong and adequately supple. (Also add this to your list: Practice good foot and toenail hygiene!)

In this chapter, I'll give you the guidelines you need to get your feet into the best possible shape—and keep them that way.

THE NATURAL FOOT

For most of our 4-million-year history, human beings roamed the earth barefoot or wore only a thin layer of animal skin wrapped around the foot as protection against the elements. Just contemplating this makes most of us want to reach down and rub our feet. But if you understand how the foot works and how it's constructed, it makes perfect sense.

To begin with, the soles of our feet contain more than 200,000 nerve endings, more than almost any other part of our body. This means that our feet are designed to be highly sensitive. The skin on the soles of our feet is also 20 times thicker than the skin on any other part of our body. This means our feet are also tough: They are built to stand up to the friction of the earth's variable terrain, and to do so over the course of a lifetime, all while taking in loads of neural information and radiating that up to the rest of our musculoskeletal system.

Think about how it feels when you walk barefoot on a sandy beach. The feeling is quite different than walking while wearing shoes. (It's great!) You can feel the tiny granules of sand between your toes, the smooth, hard tops of beach pebbles beneath the ball of your foot, and the sharp edges of shells along your instep. The truth is, walking barefoot on a beach—or anywhere else in a natural environment that isn't polluted with shards of glass, metal, or plastic—is one of the sublime pleasures of life.

When we're walking on a beach or any other natural terrain, our foot moves in wonderfully synchronized and adaptive ways—every part of the foot making contact with the ground constantly adjusts and interacts with it. This is how our feet were designed to work optimally. Bare feet on beach sand are fluid and flexible—hardly the stiff, bony body parts that we dutifully stuff into shoes or sneakers every day. Unfortunately, when we do wear shoes all the time, our bodies "forget" something essential. (And it's no wonder, given that most of us were put into our first pair of shoes before we could even walk.)

So keep in mind, your feet love being bare. Just think of the activities that require our feet to be flexible and responsive, such as yoga, swimming, gymnastics, and many forms of dance. All these activities are best performed with bare feet!

Still skeptical? The winner of the gold medal in the marathon at the 1960 Olympics was an Ethiopian runner named Abebe Bikila—and he ran the race barefoot.

PARTS OF THE FOOT

Your foot is made up of soft tissue and bones working together to form a healthy, functioning base that supports and activates much of your motion. Understanding the construction of our feet, and how they function, can go a long way in preventing and correcting foot problems.

The principal parts of the foot are the heel, instep (the high part on top of the front of your foot), sole, ball, and five toes. Whenever too much pressure is applied to any one of these areas, there is a risk of foot pain and injury. That's not to say that pressure is bad for our feet; they are designed to withstand incredible amounts of pressure. But abnormally high pressure causes most of the common types of foot pain. (As I've pointed out before, a simple walk loads your skeleton and feet with several times your body weight in pressure, while running and jumping increase this load many times over.)

ANATOMY OF THE FOOT

Anterior Talofibular Ligament

Soleus

Soleus Gastrocnemius

Tibalis Posterior

Achilles Tendon

Plantar Fascia

HOW TO NURTURE YOUR FEET

Not all feet are created equal. Some tilt in, or out, or they support your body in such a way that your weight is unevenly distributed. Way down there at foot level, those small differences in support can make a big difference in your comfort level. So it's worthwhile to take a moment and look at what's going on. Here are some things to notice:

● Standing with bare feet on a bare floor, hip width apart, feel the way your feet make contact with the floor. Now look at your feet, your ankles, and your shins. Does everything look like it is in alignment?

● Lift your toes and feel where the weight is being distributed on the floor. You should feel weight at the ball of the foot, the base of the baby toe, and the heel. Is there even weight on the front and back of your foot, or is there more in front than in back? Does your weight roll more to the inside or outside of your feet?

● Now see whether you can even out these forces. Spread your toes and think about pressing each one into the ground. Making these slight adjustments will improve your basic stance and balance.

The foot has three arches, making it a structure that is both stable when standing and flexible when in motion. The most familiar arch is the medial longitudinal arch—the one that runs from the inner heel up to the ball of the big toe. But there's also a lateral longitudinal arch running from the outer heel up to the ball of the little toe. And, finally, you have a transverse arch extending from the ball of the big toe to the base of the little toe.

Your feet are balanced when your body weight is evenly distributed over the three points of a tripod—your heel, the ball of the big toe, and the ball of the little toe. The arches connecting those points are what put a spring in our step, work as shock absorbers, and help our bodies adapt to uneven surfaces.

When you're walking, your feet are constantly changing shape in a pattern of normal foot motions called *pronation* and *supination*. You can see your feet go through these motions if you stand barefoot on a flat surface with your feet hip width apart and (without moving your feet) turn as far as you can to your right. You will feel more weight going to the outside of the foot, and the medial longitudinal arch will lift slightly. It's said that your right foot is *supinating*. At the same time, when you make that shift to the right, your left side will perform the opposite motion. The left foot goes into *pronation*, with the arch flattening and the weight moving to the inside of the foot.

As the right foot supinates, it becomes more rigid. (Supination stiffens the foot, allowing better leverage to push off on each step in walking.) The left foot, in pronation, "unlocks" and becomes a more mobile adapter to the surface beneath. Your feet are constantly going through these motions of supination and pronation every time you take a step. But of course it all happens so fast, and so instinctively, that we don't have to train our feet to do it.

THE MIRROR OF OUR HEALTH

Feet are a great indicator of our overall health. That's why many health professionals involved with feet call them the mirror of our health. The first symptoms

---

SIMPLE STRETCHES FOR YOUR FEET

Here are some gentle stretches to keep your feet healthy, strong, and flexible. All can be done in a standing position:

- Raise and curl your toes 10 times, holding each position for a count of five.

- When you walk, focus on pushing off from your toes. This strengthens the flexors of the toes.

- Regularly pick up objects from the floor with your feet—washcloths, a towel, or even pencils.

- Pump your feet up and down (mime-walk) to stretch the calf and shin muscles. This is a great exercise to do while waiting in line.

of nerve and circulatory disorders, as well as conditions such as arthritis and diabetes, commonly show up in the foot before anywhere else. In other words, a foot ailment may very well be the first sign of a more serious medical problem. (This explains why gerontologists, doctors who specialize in treating the elderly, always examine their patients' feet closely. If an elderly person has good foot hygiene and the feet are generally in good shape, it is one indicator that basic overall health is good, too.)

Your feet are the foundation for your body. All the joints above require well-functioning feet to enable you to maintain the active life that keeps you in your prime.

OUR FEET AS WE AGE

Although our feet are designed to function for a lifetime, they do change as we add on years. They become longer. The internal tissues, as well as the skin, become thinner. The fluids that keep the bones and joints of the foot operating smoothly diminish, too. Also, after years of working as spring-loaded shock absorbers, our arches begin to fall and flatten out. The foot widens, too.

While all these changes are going on in your feet as you age, there are other changes in the rest of the body that challenge the feet in new ways. Older people tend to experience more issues with balance. As the feet become more fragile, it is important for us to build stability work and balance work into our fitness programs.

Healthy feet are a must, at any age. Unless your feet are functioning well, your ligaments, joints, and muscles will not work as they should. That's why it's so crucial to make foot health a cornerstone in our desire to be prime for life.

OH, MY ACHING FEET: COMMON AILMENTS

Very few of us are born with foot problems, but sooner or later many of us are forced to deal with any number of them. Most foot ailments are caused by too much stress being placed on a specific part of the foot. Here are some of the most common (and painful!) foot ailments reported today.

Plantar Fasciitis

This is a straining, tearing, or degeneration of the plantar fascia, the band of tissue that starts at the heel and runs along the bottom of the foot. That tissue attaches to each of the bones that form the transverse arch. The plantar fascia, with ligaments that act like rubber bands between the bones in the foot, helps form the main arch in your foot. When you bend your toes up, the tissue becomes tighter and lifts the arch higher, stiffening the entire foot for leverage when you push off your foot while walking.

There is a pad of fat under your heel that protects the end of the plantar fascia, and this helps absorb the shock your heel takes when you walk. Damage to the plantar fascia causes heel pain that, left untreated, can radiate through the entire length of the tissue.

As we age, the plantar fascia loses some of its elasticity, and the fat pad on the heel begins to thin. This reduces the shock-absorbing capabilities of the heel and may lead to the plantar fascia becoming bruised or torn. Other risk factors for developing plantar fasciitis (inflammation of the plantar fascia) include being overweight, having diabetes, spending most of the day on your feet, becoming very active in a short amount of time (i.e., intensive training for a sporting event), and having either a high arch or a flat foot. If you have plantar fasciitis, the discomfort is usually worse first thing in the morning, especially when your feet first hit the floor.

If You Have the Symptoms Above . . .

If you discovered in Chapter 3 that you have short, stiff gastrocnemius and soleus muscles, your feet may benefit from those stretches, especially if you make the following modification: Place a rolled washcloth under the arch of your bare foot in back, and another under your big toe to hold it a little off the floor as you do these stretches. This *gently* stretches the plantar fascia. *Go easy*. Repeat this several times and do it four to six times per day, if possible.

Sometimes stretching alone isn't enough. As with any chronic pain, taking over-the-counter pain remedies such as ibuprofen (Advil), acetaminophen (Tylenol), or naproxen (Aleve) may help. The use of orthotic inserts (orthoses) can also help. (See page 110 for some advice on how to choose orthoses.)

Joan's
STORY

Joan, one of my clients at Canyon Ranch, had a pretty severe case of plantar fasciitis when she arrived. She had made the mistake of thinking that, if she worked out hard for several weeks before she got to the Ranch, she'd get more out of her experience there. Unfortunately, all she did was strain the plantar fascia in her right foot.

I saw the problem when I first examined Joan's foot and ankle. I asked her to walk across the room and watched her limp along on her shortened calf muscles. Ouch! I took a pair of soft, inexpensive over-the-counter orthotic inserts made of foam from my desk and tucked them into her shoes. Then I asked her to walk again.

"That's a bit better," she told me, "but there are a couple of spots where it's poking my foot."

She sat down. I took the insoles from her and made a few adjustments, simply sanding down the high points with sandpaper. Then she tried them again.

"Better still." She actually managed to smile.

I explained to Joan how the orthotic insert actually helped her foot. In part, plantar fasciitis is an inability of the foot to absorb the shock of landing and standing. So a soft, inexpensive orthotic device simply spreads the force of the body weight over a larger surface area, and thus decreasing the stress to the plantar fascia. But, I emphasized, this was only for temporary relief and did not address the overall underlying cause. The cause was that her calves were too short and too stiff. I gave Joan the soleus and gastrocnemius stretches, adding the suggestion to prop up her big toes and arches with washcloths as she was doing these stretches. By the time she left Canyon Ranch, she was feeling almost 100 percent!

GOOD ORTHOSES THAT ANYONE CAN AFFORD

Most people do not need orthotic devices to have healthy, comfortable feet. Interestingly, research has shown that inexpensive, over-the-counter orthoses can be as effective as expensive custom ones. And there's a considerable advantage in price. Custom orthoses can range in cost from $200 to $1,000 a pair, while over-the-counter orthoses are generally in the range of $10 to $30.

Here are some specific over-the-counter recommendations:

● Try Superfeet, Birkenstock, Dr. Scholl's, or New Balance orthoses. (The ones made by New Balance, however, may only fit their brand of shoes.) AliMed (800-225-2610) makes an excellent pair called Freedom XPE that cost $15 to $20; no prescription is necessary. When you try out the orthoses with athletic shoes, just slip them in the shoe under the removable sock liner.

● If you can test shoes right in the store, do so. Ideally, you want to walk around at your normal pace for 20 minutes or so. If they feel comfortable afterward, that's a good indication of a successful fit. (This is not rocket science, obviously. You just want orthoses that give your foot more contact with the bottom of the shoe, to disperse force and increase comfort.)

● A therapist or pedorthist may also alter them with a heat gun or by adding some inexpensive materials. The experts at making orthoses and altering them are often not the doctors or therapists but, rather, the pedorthists who are experts at working with the materials.

Tips for Minimizing the Pain of Plantar Fasciitis

For clients like Joan who come to us with foot pain, I recommend these simple steps to help alleviate the pain before we start a stretching plan.

○ Cut back on all the weight–bearing activities that you can— including walking. Rest is essential for the tissue to heal.

○ Wear shoes that have a soft, orthopedically designed foot bed such as Birkenstocks or Mephistos, rather than shoes with stiff soles, including rigid athletic shoes.

○ Avoid spending time barefoot until the pain is gone.

○ Before you rise from bed in the morning, sit on the edge of the mattress. Cross your right foot at the ankle over your left knee. Take your right foot in your hands and gently pull the toes back or up with your right hand. Gently knead the arch of your right foot with the knuckles of your left hand. (Or you can roll it across a rolling pin on the floor.) This gently stretches the fascia. Then treat the left foot the same way. When you're done, get in the shower and close the drain. Let the warm, soothing water cover your feet.

○ Talk to your physical therapist or doctor about night splints. These keep your feet in proper alignment while you sleep, so that your calf muscles stay long and flexible.

○ If you've been wearing high heels, stiff boots, or dress shoes, put them in the closet and leave them there. If you need to wear a structured shoe, athletic shoes are best, especially if you have flat feet with the arch low to the ground. Comfort is the most important consideration.

○ Individuals with very flexible joints who do not have short or stiff calf muscles are also prone to plantar fasciitis. Soft or semirigid orthoses to disperse pressure over a larger surface area help these individuals, too. Although the traditional approach for flat, flexible feet like this is to use rigid plastic orthoses, I usually recommend softer, yielding ones. They work well and are much more comfortable.

A SPRAINED ANKLE

Sprained ankles are fairly common and can be very painful and debilitating. Most sprained ankles involve the ligaments on the outside of the ankle and are called "inversion" sprains. These sprains occur, often, when we lose our footing, and

ANKLE RESCUE

If you have a sprained ankle, early attention from a doctor or physical therapist could help you recover a lot more quickly than you would otherwise. Not all ankle sprains respond to the Mulligan technique (see opposite page), but it can quickly and dramatically help in many cases. It can also prevent recurrent sprains.

Should you see a physical therapist *before* you see a doctor? You do have a choice. Most states allow you to see a physical therapist without a doctor's referral. Many physicians don't know about practices such as the Mulligan technique because it is a physical therapy technique. Because of this, it can make a big difference to see a physical therapist for ankle sprains as soon as possible. If you have had recurring sprains, it may especially benefit you to seek the help of a physical therapist who can analyze some of the movements or weaknesses that could be contributing to the problem.

To find a physical therapist for manual therapy treatment of foot problems:

- Go to www.apta.org.

- Click on "Professional Development," then "Find a Certified Specialist."

- Then click on "View the Directory."

- Under "Specialty Area," click and drag in the drag-down menu to select "Orthopaedic."

- For "Practice Focus," select either "Foot and Ankle" or "Manual Therapy."

This same Web site lists the states where you are allowed to see a physical therapist without a doctor's referral.

the ligaments get stretched too far. As a result, there is usually a lot of swelling and stiffness at the site of the sprain.

Prevention of Sprained Ankles

Ankle sprains are correlated with an incorrect perception of where your body is in space. Balance exercises help correct this.

Harriet's
STORY

Harriet was a guest at the Ranch who, unfortunately, had stepped into a pothole when she was on her way to the airport for her "week of rest and relaxation." When I met her, her ankle was quite swollen. I asked Harriet if she'd let me try a technique that involves gently manipulating the outside anklebone in an inversion sprain and moving it back into place. This procedure, called the Mulligan technique, is named for a New Zealand physical therapist who realized that sometimes in an inversion sprain the anklebone moves a bit out of place, causing pain and swelling.

I assured Harriet that though the Mulligan technique sounded painful, it wasn't. She agreed she'd like me to give it a try. Using my hands, I gently pressed on her anklebone, coaxing it to settle back into its correct position with tiny oscillations. I asked Harriet to let me know right away if she felt any pain. After about 5 minutes of this, I asked her to stand up. Immediately, there was much less swelling. Harriet told me that the pain had also decreased noticeably. I taped her ankle to provide additional support.

The next day, we started a regime of gentle exercises to improve her circulation and strengthen the muscles and ligaments in her ankle and foot. By the end of the week, her ankle was almost back to normal.

○ Keeping the muscles on the outside of the hip strong may have an enormous influence on preventing sprained ankles. Weakness of the gluteus medius has been linked to inversions of the ankle. Faulty hip control causes faulty foot placement and instability of the entire lower extremity. Perform the gluteus medius strength exercise explained in this book (page 80).

THE *RICE* TREATMENT

RICE is the acronym for Rest, Ice, Compression, and Elevation. This is the protocol of choice immediately following many kinds of joint injuries. Here are the components:

Rest: Reduce your activity until the swelling and pain subside, usually 3 or 4 days. Avoid activities that cause pain. Do not return to the activity that caused the problem until your PT or physician advises you that it is safe to do so. It is usually recommended you return to activities that caused the injury *gradually* and stop if pain occurs.

Ice: Apply ice wrapped in cloth every 15 minutes per hour the first day, then every 3 to 4 hours for the second and third days. Be cautious, however: Leaving the ice on for more than 20 minutes can cause frostbite. (Moist cold—applying a wet towel between the skin and the ice pack—penetrates more deeply and quickly than dry cold does.)

Compression: Wrapping the joint in an ACE bandage (elastic bandage) can limit swelling and relieve pain. But if the area below the wrap becomes colder than the other leg, it means the bandage is too tight. Be sure to keep it loose enough. And always remove the wrap before bedtime.

Elevation: Elevate the joint above the level of the heart (place on a pillow) while icing to further reduce inflammation.

If the condition is mild, RICE may be enough treatment. For many injuries, however, this is just a starting point. Some physical therapy is beneficial as well.

○ Another method is balance training. Here's how it's done:

1. Stand on one leg and balance for up to 1 minute. If you're unsteady, practice in an empty closet (using the walls to catch yourself if you start to tip), or stand with your hands hovering above a solid countertop. If you have a very solid, heavy, high-backed chair, you can also stand near that for safety.

2. When you can balance for 1 minute, try standing on one leg with your eyes closed. You'll feel your lower leg muscles

stabilizing you with sway control. Your muscles get an excellent workout, and that strengthens your ankle. (One caution, however: If you've sprained an ankle before, you'll probably be more unsteady when you put weight on the ankle that was injured.)

Treatment for Sprained Ankles

For a diagnosis, and to rule out the possibility that you've fractured your ankle (which would require an entirely different therapy), be sure to see a physical therapist or physician as soon as possible after you've sprained your ankle. As long as you don't have a fracture or some other injury, you can probably begin with the RICE treatment (described in the sidebar on the opposite page). In addition, here are some other steps I'd recommend.

○ Make alphabet letters with your foot, inscribing them in the air. Make them as large as you can without pain. This exercises all the muscles in the foot and ankle. To be painless, the movements may need to be minuscule. (If you experience discomfort, don't do this exercise.)

○ Several times per day, with your leg and foot elevated on a bunch of pillows, for several minutes, pump your foot as though you were pushing up and down on a gas pedal. This literally helps pump fluid up out of the region to help decrease swelling. (Again, stop at once if you begin to feel any pain.)

○ Get mobile quickly. The faster you get any tissue moving, the faster it tends to heal—as long as there's no pain. Sometimes, you may need to use crutches to keep your weight off the ankle. Go ahead and use them if it means you stay moving.

○ Most people can return to bicycling very quickly, because that motion places little stress on the outside of the ankle. Swimming is fine, too—the water pressure can actually decrease swelling—but be careful about pushing off the wall too hard or putting too much weight on your foot in the shallow end. Again, avoid pain.

○ Return to walking or running on flat terrain only when totally pain free. Add uneven terrain, turning, and cutting movements very gently and gradually.

○ Ice, typically recommended for the acute phase of the first few weeks, can be helpful for months afterward in helping to prevent swelling. Following injury, apply ice or a cold pack any time you do an activity that "challenges" your ankle. Just be sure to follow the standard cautions: Wrap the ice in a towel and don't apply it more than 15 minutes in order to avoid frostbite.

Achilles Tendon Problems

We've all heard the Greek myth of Achilles, considered to be the bravest hero in the Trojan War. When Achilles was born, his mother, Thetis, tried to make him immortal by dipping him in the river Styx. As she immersed him, she held him by one heel. Alas, she forgot to dip him again to cover the heel where she'd held him. This one spot, on the back of Achilles' foot, was the only place on his body where he was mortal and vulnerable. Achilles fought heroically against the Trojans, but Paris killed him when an arrow pierced the area that will forever be known as the "Achilles heel."

Actually, when we refer to the Achilles heel, we're talking about a tendon. It's the strong tendon that connects the muscles of the calf with the heel bone. That's the point of vulnerability.

Injuring your Achilles tendon is not only painful, but it can also lead to serious long-term problems if not treated aggressively and quickly. The Achilles tendon is the largest tendon in the body, and if it ruptures, it makes walking virtually impossible: The muscles of the outer calf are no longer attached to the foot.

There are certain conditions that increase the risk of injury to the Achilles tendon, including high blood pressure, diabetes, and obesity. See a physician or physical therapist for guidance if you have any of these conditions. If you are experiencing Achilles tendonosis (a degeneration of the tendon) and there is no rupture, you'll want to pay a visit to a physical therapist. He or she may prescribe a series of what are called "eccentric strength-training exercises" that can help the tendon mend.

For Prevention of Achilles Tendon Problems, Try This:

○ Stand on the edge of a step with your heels just off the edge, holding the railing for support.

○ Rise up onto the balls of both feet, and then slowly lower your heels down until you feel a slight stretch in your Achilles tendon.

○ Time your movements so that you rise for 2 seconds, and then lower yourself for 4 to 6 seconds. Repeat 8 to 15 times. Then rest for 1 minute.

○ Do this exercise 3 nonconsecutive days per week, performing two or three sets of 8 to 15 repetitions. If you do multiple sets, be sure to allow a minute's rest between each one.

○ To increase strength in the tendon, when you can do three sets of 15 repetitions, put a knapsack on your shoulders with 5 pounds of weight in it. Or you can hold something weighing 5 pounds in one hand. Over time, keep adding to the weight in 5-pound increments. In other words, when you can do three sets of 15 repetitions with a given resistance (or amount of weight), you're ready to add another 5 pounds.

This eccentric strength-training exercise challenges the muscles at the end of the tendons and strengthens the tendon itself. Because of that, you may experience some initial soreness, but this is normal. Repeat and the soreness should go away after 3 or 4 days, as long as you continue on a regular basis.

Bunions

You have a bunion (hallux valgus) when your big toe begins to point toward the outside of the foot, angling toward the baby toe. Bunions come on gradually over the years. They tend to run in families, and women have a significantly higher incidence of bunions than men do.

For many years, it was thought that wearing shoes that were too tight caused bunions. When the toes are compressed into the point of a shoe, it pushes the big toe laterally. Although it's true that wearing tight shoes is indeed a risk factor, there may be other causes as well. A severely pronating foot—that is, a foot that constantly rolls heel in as you walk—may also tend to push the big toe out of alignment.

Yet another factor can be weak hip abductors, particularly the back of the gluteus medius. This muscle's main function is to prevent the knee from dropping into the midline (hip adduction) when standing, sitting, going up and down steps, or walking on uneven terrain.

If that muscle isn't strong enough to do this, your feet may pronate slightly every time you take a step, pushing the big toe out toward your other toes.

Treatment for Bunions

Most bunions don't hurt when you're just walking along, but you may feel a lot of pain if the big toe is bent upward. They can also disrupt your fitness program. Try these remedies for relief:

○ Wear stiff-soled shoes such as clogs. These take stress off the first metatarsal joints, including that of the big toe, so you'll be more comfortable. Or ask for rocker sole shoes at a specialty shoe store.

○ Visit a podiatrist, pedorthist, or physical therapist who specializes in feet and ankles for assistance. These foot specialists can help make shoe adjustments, using a small, fabricated wedge that's placed under and across the width of the sole of your shoe behind the toes. The wedge diminishes toe extension.

FINDING ROCKER SOLE SHOES

A rocker sole shoe has a stiff, rounded bottom and doesn't bend much under the toes. Instead, in this type of shoe, you tend to roll across the bottom of the shoe and the bunion receives less stress.

To find this shoe, you might need to look in stores that specialize in foot problems. The MBT, Swiss Masai shoe (www.swissmasaius.com) is an extreme example of a rocker sole shoe. (There are other, cheaper shoes with rocker soles that will also help.) They are not necessarily miracle shoes, as advertised, but with some foot problems such as bunions, they can help. The extreme rocker sole does perturb balance significantly, so if you have severe balance problems, test them in the store.

LIFTING THE ARCH OF YOUR FOOT

If you were asked to increase the arch of your foot, the first thing you'd probably do is turn your toes under so you get more lift. But when you do that, you're not testing or exercising the posterior tibialis tendon, which is the one responsible for maintaining your arch. Strong muscles in the longitudinal arch can help prevent plantar fasciitis and other common foot problems.

It may take some patient practice before you can put that tendon to work, but here's the way to do it:

- Place your bare foot on a smooth, hard floor. Relax the muscles under the longitudinal arch (i.e., allow the arch to relax and drop).

- Now, try to pull in the arch, shortening it. This will lift the arch. But don't flex or pull the toes under; they must remain relaxed. Only the muscles within the arch should contract.

At first, it may be nearly impossible to detect the difference between the position of the relaxed arch and the lifted arch. But if you practice this frequently, it will become easier.

When you can, practice standing on the "short foot" while lifting the other foot off the floor. Build up gradually in duration to 1 minute per side. Eventually, try doing this with your eyes closed.

Interdigital Neuromas

Neuromas are growths in the nerves that run between your toes. Chronic stress on these nerves causes swelling and pain. Again, this could be the result of wearing shoes with a tight toe box. When toes are pressed tightly against each other, it compresses the nerves between them.

Treatment for Interdigital Neuromas

○ Avoid wearing tight shoes.

○ See a foot-care specialist (podiatrist, pedorthist, or physical therapist) to be fitted with a metatarsal pad. This is a small, dome-shaped pad that is placed under and just behind the heads of the toes. It spreads the toes apart, often eliminating pain.

○ Corticosteroids help some patients. (This medication alleviates symptoms but may not eliminate the cause of the problem, which is mechanical compression of the nerve.) You'll need to see a doctor for these injections.

Flat Feet

When you sit or stand, can you lift your arch without pulling your toes under? Some people have a very difficult time doing this. To raise the height of the arch, you need to use a muscle called the posterior tibialis.

If it's been overstretched from years of having a flat, flexible arch, the posterior tibialis can become weak, and you'll lose the ability to hold up your arch. The bones of your mid-foot start bulging inward, and your arch becomes very flat. Your posterior tibialis tendon becomes inflamed and painful. You'll feel this pain just behind your inside anklebone, and below and around it.

(In a worst-case scenario, your tendon may rupture. At this point, you have "adult acquired flat foot." It's a painful condition that may require surgery—a fusion of the rear foot bones.)

There are many ways to help prevent posterior tibialis strain. You can fit yourself with orthoses that prevent the arch from being chronically overstretched. Do strength training to improve the function of the posterior tibialis. (See the sidebar on page 119, "Lifting the Arch of Your Foot.") And wear shoes that control the mid-foot: Lace-up shoes are a necessity!

If you have flat feet, you definitely need to see a podiatrist or physical therapist who focuses on the foot.

ESSENTIAL WAYS TO PREVENT FOOT PAIN

If you have excessive pronation and hypermobile foot joints, there are at least two ways to enjoy pain-free activity. With the right orthoses, or a change to better-fitting shoes, or both, there's a good chance you can resume pleasurable activity.

Prevention is everything. Avoid activities that cause pain in your feet. If you just cannot seem to get rid of foot pain, here's what I recommend:

- It's important to see your doctor, a podiatrist (foot specialist), or a physical therapist who specializes in the foot immediately.

- Inspect your feet regularly. Look for any changes in coloration, temperature, or texture of the skin. Look for thick or discolored nails (a possible sign of fungus growth) and check for cracks or cuts in the skin, especially if you have diabetes.

- Wash your feet often, especially between the toes, and be sure to dry them well before putting on socks or shoes. If you get dry skin, use foot cream to prevent blisters.

- Trim your toenails straight across and not too short. (Cutting nails at the corners may cause ingrown toenails.)

- Make sure your shoes fit properly.

- Alternate shoes: Don't wear the same pair of shoes every day. It's important to expose your foot to different foot beds to keep them supple and flexible. Running or walking shoes have decreased shock absorption for up to 24 hours after an hour of wear, so alternating two pairs can help your feet.

- Be cautious using home remedies on your feet. Improper treatment can turn a minor problem into a major one.

- If you have diabetes, have a podiatrist check your feet at *least* once a year. People with diabetes or heart problems are far more prone to foot infections than others. Due to nerve damage and impaired bloodflow, they often lose sensation in their feet.

10 STEPS TO CHOOSING THE PERFECT SHOE

It's ironic that shoes, which were created to protect our feet, have become so harmful to them! But it doesn't have to be that way if you choose your shoes with care. Research has shown that comfort is the best determinant of shoe or orthotic fit. Trust your feel. Choose footwear that feels good.

Here are 10 helpful tips for buying shoes:

1. Always buy shoes from a shop with a large selection of shoes and a well-trained staff.

2. Get your feet measured every time you purchase a shoe. An adult's foot may change sizes four or five times during a lifetime. Also, a "standard size" shoe may not always correspond to your foot. So when you're trying them on, focus on comfort rather than size. And avoid high heels!

3. Shop for shoes late in the day, when your feet are at their largest. (Feet swell when you've been doing a lot of standing around.)

4. Look for the ideal shoe. It has a broad-based, low heel and adequate toe box (so your toes don't feel cramped). The sole should be flat and flexible. And you want a shoe that is made of lightweight, breathable, and flexible material. These qualities are what make leather ideal.

5. If you have osteoarthritis in your feet, knees, or hips, make sure that you choose shoes that have adequate shock absorption in the midsoles.

6. If you have a narrow foot, you need to make sure the shoelaces will hold your foot in place when they're pulled tight. (A lacing pattern called "lock lacing" helps prevent heel slippage.) If this doesn't help, buy shoes with a narrower heel.

7. When trying on shoes, be alert to any pain on the forefoot or tingling in the toes. There is a nerve running down the top of your foot, and if the lacing over that nerve is too tight, it can cause the pain or tingling. If you have a high instep, you're especially prone to this problem. To eliminate pressure, you can try a lacing pattern called "bow-tie lacing." This eliminates pressure.

8. When you try on shoes, choose the one that fits your larger foot. Walk around the store with the shoes on, take your time, and don't buy them if they're not comfortable. Shoes never "break in"—our feet do. Most good shoe stores will let you return them if you only wear them inside once. Some running shoe stores have treadmills to let you "test ride" them for 15 to 20 minutes.

9. Buy shoes with adjustable fastenings, such as those with laces, straps, or Velcro. Being able to fit the shoe properly to the shape of your foot is vital. Your foot should not slip when it is in a properly fitting shoe.

10. Whenever you can, take off your shoes and stretch your feet. Let them make contact with the earth as they were designed to do! Treat them lovingly and kindly: The health of your feet is crucial.

A SOURCE OF LACING TECHNIQUES

Ian's Shoelace Site is an excellent Web site that shows many lace-up techniques. If you wear lace-up shoes, you'll want to check out this site to find what's most comfortable for you. Here's the address: www.fieggen.com/shoelace/index.htm.

CHAPTER SEVEN

THE KNEE

"Have you noticed that whatever sport
you're trying to learn, some earnest person
is always telling you to keep your knees
bent?"

—*Dave Barry*

"When a batter swings and I see his
knees move, I can tell what his weaknesses
are, and then I just put the ball where I
know he can't hit it."

—*Satchel Paige*

Nothing is more demoralizing than suffering from knee pain. It can make the most physically fit person feel a million years old. This kind of pain, unfortunately, is quite common, but it's not because our knees are poorly designed, per se; it's more about the unreasonable things we often expect them to do, plus the punishment we give them.

If you are or have ever been an athlete, you've likely been told by a coach how poorly designed and injury prone the knee is. That somehow, if you push yourself hard enough, you'll manage to perform *in spite* of this primitive body part. Well, that's just a load of hogwash. It is true that the knee is highly prone to injury, but that's because of its incredible complexity and the extraordinary—and sometimes unreasonable—things we expect of it.

As with any joint, taking measures to prevent pain and injury are your best strategies. If you've never experienced knee pain, you are among the lucky few, and I will provide tips and exercises in this chapter that will keep you pain free. If you already have trouble with your knees, don't despair; you can and will find your way back to knee health and get back on the path to being prime for life.

If you start to feel the slightest twinge of discomfort in your knees, try a few simple things right away:

○ Avoid all pain and activities that encourage excessive twisting.

○ When you exercise, make sure that everything you do feels easy on your knees.

○ When you're walking or running, lead with your feet; don't advance your knees out over your toes.

○ When you go from a bent-knee to a straight-knee position, don't allow your knees to snap back.

○ Wear the right shoes. (If your knees begin to hurt when you wear certain shoes, put them away for good.)

○ Honor your knee's alignment—keep your thighs in line with your feet.

Physical therapists treat musculoskeletal problems with a different perspective than orthopedic surgeons do. The physician is an expert at medical diagnoses and surgical treatments of knee issues. We physical therapists are movement diagnosticians—experts at diagnosing and correcting movement problems. Our diagnosis reflects function and movement. This chapter will give you some understanding of common medical diagnoses and a physical therapist's perspective on treatment for the most common functional diagnoses that I encounter.

Based on years of experience as a physical therapist, I know that knee injuries are all too common. And that's why a little knowledge of physiology comes in handy; if you understand how things work and how they can get off track, you can take the right preventive measures and keep your knees pain and injury free.

A CLOSER LOOK AT THE KNEE

Your knee is actually the largest joint in your body, the place where your major leg bones, and their attendant muscles and ligaments, intersect. The knee is made up of the lower end of the thighbone (the femur) and the upper end of your shinbone (the tibia). The tip of the fibula (the bone that runs along the side of the shin) is connected to the same region, but is functionally a part of your ankle. Protecting these bones is the kneecap (the patella), and the whole structure is held together and supported by an intricate network of ligaments and tendons and muscle.

- Your kneecap slides in a groove on the end of your femur.

- The kneecap acts like a pulley to increase the strength of your quadriceps, the muscles on the front of your thigh.

- The surfaces where the bones in your knee touch are covered with smooth cartilage—called articular cartilage. This pearly, smooth cartilage is 65 to 75 percent fluid and is a shock-absorbing surface. Receiving no bloodflow, it requires movement of loading and unloading to bring nutrients in and waste products out.

- The surfaces inside your knee joint are lubricated with synovial fluid.

The knee is what's known as a hinge joint, an apparatus specifically designed to swing back and forth freely, but not to move too much laterally (side to side). It does have some ability to rotate or twist, too. Aside from its central role in facilitating the movement of the leg, it also supports nearly all of your body weight. Because of these roles, it is the joint that is most susceptible to acute injury and to the development of osteoarthritis, which is the result of erosion of the articular cartilage.

In day-to-day life, our knees function without too much stress put on them. Walking, climbing, and squatting are motions that knees are perfectly designed to handle. But throw in anything that stresses this hinge (think of the lateral load put on your knee if you ski or—ouch!—the hit a professional running back takes to the side of his body when slammed by a hard-charging linebacker) and the knee is put at serious risk. The ligaments and tendons are easily damaged when

ANATOMY OF THE KNEE

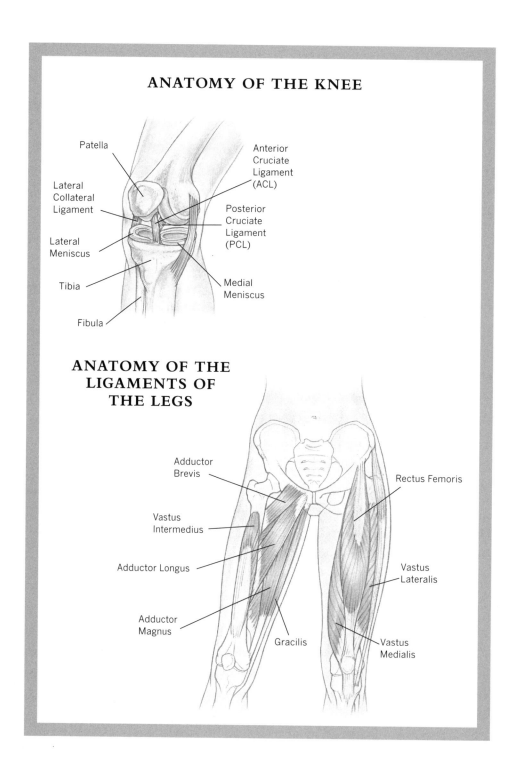

Patella

Anterior
Cruciate
Ligament
(ACL)

Lateral
Collateral
Ligament

Posterior
Cruciate
Ligament
(PCL)

Lateral
Meniscus

Tibia

Medial
Meniscus

Fibula

ANATOMY OF THE LIGAMENTS OF THE LEGS

Adductor
Brevis

Rectus Femoris

Vastus
Intermedius

Adductor Longus

Vastus
Lateralis

Adductor
Magnus

Gracilis

Vastus
Medialis

stressed unnaturally, as are the menisci and other soft tissues. These tissues, such as cartilage, help cushion and lubricate the joint.

Knee surgery is the number one type of orthopedic operation performed in the world today.

KNEE SURGERY

Research is equivocal regarding whether surgery is better in the long run than conservative care (i.e., physical therapy and no surgery). The few number of studies have shown that both provide good long-term outcomes in most patients. Surgery patients tend to have a higher incidence of other medical complications (risks of surgery), but conservatively treated patients tend to undergo slightly more subsequent surgeries. Again, it probably depends on what is expected of the knee. Running and cutting sports require the necessary stability of an intact (or repaired) anterior cruciate ligament (ACL).

The Ligaments

There are four ligaments (see the illustrations to the left) that help stabilize the knee. These are taut ropes of connective tissue that hold the joint in position, and they limit how far the bones of the knee (meaning the tibia and femur) can move. Ligaments protect the knee joint from becoming dislocated. The two cruciate (anterior and posterior) ligaments cross one another on the inside of the knee joint and limit front-to-back motion. The two collateral ligaments are outside the knee joint, and they're the ones that limit side-to-side motion.

The cruciate ligaments, which are on the inside of the knee, can rarely heal on their own because they lack an adequate blood supply and are bathed in joint fluid. Because of this, surgery is often the only option for any sustained improvement. (Strengthening the leg can offer a reduction in pain but will not restore proper knee function for performing turning, cutting activities such as skiing, dancing, or playing soccer.)

Is surgery necessary? For many people, the answer depends on what their knees are expected to do. For full stability, surgery is necessary, but it carries an increased risk of osteoarthritis later in life. Each trauma adds to the risk. But there are many adults who want to be fit and healthy and are willing to forego extreme sports. With strengthening, their knees may function fine without surgery. (I'll talk more about specific ligament injuries later in this chapter.)

The Menisci

In the illustration, you can see that the menisci (plural of meniscus) are crescent-shaped pieces of cartilage wedged between the bones (tibia and femur) that meet behind the kneecap (patella). This cartilage acts as a "spacer," having the primary job of spreading the force of the two bony ends of the femur (and all of your upper body weight) onto the joint surface of the tibia. Your menisci protect the articular cartilage on the bony ends from wear and tear. A torn meniscus is common for people over 40.

THE AGING KNEE: OSTEOARTHRITIS

Inevitably, our knees, like the rest of our bodies, begin to show the signs of a lifetime of use. The most common symptom of an aging knee is the onset of osteoarthritis (sometimes called the "wear and tear" arthritis), which sets in when the articular cartilage wear away. As I've mentioned, articular cartilage has an optimal zone of physical stress. If there's no stress at all (as with someone who is paraplegic), cartilage may decrease by as much as 25 percent in 1 year. Conversely, the heaviest 20 percent of Americans demonstrate what happens when body weight puts way too much stress on that knee joint. This group has 7 to 10 times the risk of osteoarthritis. But if you're between these extremes—as most of us are—your knees may get damaged if there's excessive stress. That could come from twisting, either when you make the wrong kind of movement or when you play sports that involve a lot of turning or quick stops. Risks also include a trauma or prior surgery. This painful condition happens when the cartilage lining on the ends of bones gradually wears away.

Many guests who come to Canyon Ranch have, at one time or another, suffered a pretty serious knee injury. I see a lot of scars from all types of knee surgeries and hear many war stories from former pro athletes and overzealous weekend warriors. Most commonly, though, I see middle-aged people who never had a trauma, but come to me with aches and pains and maybe a diagnosis of osteoarthritis or a meniscal tear. Their knee is getting in the way of their joy of life. What helps these guests, or anyone interested in protecting their knees, is understanding how the knee works and what they can do to improve function and comfort.

FIVE TRUTHS ABOUT OSTEOARTHRITIS IN THE KNEE

1. Osteoarthritis can affect one or both knees.

2. There is a notoriously poor relationship between the level of arthritis one has and the amount of pain. Some individuals with severe osteoarthritis have little pain and some, with little evidence of osteoarthritis, feel a lot of pain. Pain and progression of osteoarthritis are related to misalignments. One study found that knock-kneed and bow-legged people had a faster progression of symptoms and osteoarthritis worsening.

3. If you do have osteoarthritis, you may experience pain when standing or going up and down stairs. The knee may buckle and give way, lock in place, or become stiff and swollen. These symptoms, however, could indicate many other types of knee problems.

4. Most people with osteoarthritis of the knee are over age 55 and/or obese and/or have a family history of osteoarthritis. Younger, highly active people may also develop osteoarthritis if their knee has suffered a significant injury.

5. A common misalignment that greatly exacerbates symptoms is twisting of the knee. Standing and sitting with knees twisting in or out, even slightly, can make an enormous difference to symptoms. (Going up and down steps magnifies this, too.) Focus on always aligning your thigh with your shoelaces. If you can correct twisting misalignments, you can, usually, dramatically decrease pain. Remember, it is not the arthritis that takes you to the doctor, but the pain.

TIBIOFEMORAL ROTATION SYNDROME

Knowing that the knee is the point of connection for both the shin and the thigh, it makes sense that the muscles of these parts of the leg would have to be strong in order to best support and protect the knee.

Ken's
STORY

Ken, a man in his early fifties, came to the Ranch to restore balance to his life, and this included adding the right kind of fitness to his routine. Ken had been a serious athlete when he was young. So serious that he went to college on a football scholarship and spent 4 years tearing up the football field—and his knees. By the time he was 22 years old, his football career was over. He'd had several knee surgeries to repair torn ligaments, and by age 47 he was suffering from osteoarthritis.

He channeled all of his competitive energy into other endeavors. He became a successful dentist with a big practice and was an active, hands-on father to his four kids. But in the meantime he had neglected his health by giving up regular exercise, which in turn had led him to gain 30 pounds. He also had high blood pressure and some issues with elevated blood sugar levels, and he walked with a slight limp. As he looked ahead to becoming a grandfather in the coming years, he realized that if he didn't change his lifestyle, he might miss out on doing a lot of things with his grandchildren.

When we sat down together, I asked him what his goals were. "Well," he shook his head, "I'm obviously not ever going to play full-out sports, but I'd like to lose some weight and get fit again."

Ken stayed at the Ranch for 2 weeks. Among other things, I tested his muscles for strength, range of motion, and movement. His quadriceps muscles were strong. I also tested other muscle strength and found that his hip abductor muscles on the side of his hips were very weak. The range of motion for the knee was fine, but when I asked him to walk up a single step, I noticed that he dropped his knees in toward the midline.

"That hurts!" he exclaimed. Even as he said it, I could see how his knee was twisting. So I asked him to replicate the movement with correct alignment, keeping his thigh exactly in line with his foot. "That doesn't hurt at all!" he marveled.

I asked Ken to sit down. Again, he noted the right knee hurt, and I could see it twist inward. I scratched my head.

"Ken, why didn't you keep your knee aligned correctly the way I showed you?"

He shook his head and cracked a joke. He was surprised to discover that he was literally causing his own knee pain all day. Every time he went up and down stairs, sat down and stood up, he unnecessarily twisted his knees in, and he was paying for it in terms of pain.

"My doctor told me the problem was the extra 30 pounds I gained since my football days," he said.

"So, you've got the misalignment and extra weight," I told him. "Let's figure out what we can do about it."

I explained that the tibiofemoral joint, which lies between the tibia and femur, tolerates twisting less and less well as we age. Both kinds of cartilage, meniscus and articular, don't do very well if the twisting is extreme. And then I reminded him that, now, he was aware of what he had to do. Ken had the power to stop the misalignments and significantly help his knee.

We put a plan in place. I asked him to start being aware of the times he twisted when going up and down steps, sitting, and standing. He promised he would avoid that motion. I had him work on his endurance using a stationary bicycle, activating the muscles of the front and back of his thighs, to build endurance and burn calories.

Ken discovered he still liked lifting weights, but he was to avoid the leg extension and leg curl machines in favor of a leg press and calf raise. I handed him an elastic ring (Xering) and showed him how to strengthen his weak gluteus medius muscles.

When he commented, "I thought this was a muscle only women worked on to catch our eye," I explained that strengthening these muscles would help him resist the twisting in of his knees.

Ken also was given upper body strength exercises and exercises for strengthening his midsection. He still wasn't ready for activities involving turning or twisting. He promised to avoid all movements that caused pain. Life was going to change.

At the end of the week, Ken couldn't believe the difference. And he'd been a diligent student. He reported that his pain had almost totally disappeared as long as he avoided those twisting motions. "I thought I'd need surgery," he confessed. I told him that his orthopedist was always available if he needed that—as a last resort.

Ken was able to perform squats pain free, so I sent him home armed with a set of elastic tubes and a set of exercises to get into great shape—ones that didn't obligate him to join a gym.

"Aren't squats bad for knees?" he asked me at one point. I told him that only squats done incorrectly were bad for knees and that pain would tell him whether he did them correctly. I added that it is a highly effective exercise that is also functional. It is nothing more than sitting and standing—a necessity for living.

During his stay at Canyon Ranch, Ken had also come to love the stationary bike. Now he planned to buy one to use at home. He felt that it had made the biggest difference.

I saw Ken 6 months later. He had lost 10 pounds and he looked stronger. He'd started swimming every other day (between cycling). Conscientious about avoiding the knee misalignment that had caused him so much pain, he said he avoided any strokes that might twist his knee, such as the breaststroke. He was pain free and feeling great.

Ken was typical of knee patients that I see at Canyon Ranch. My methods are simple and usually very effective. I avoid going to any pain and try to maximize function.

Seven Exercises for Tibiofemoral Syndrome

Until recently, it was presumed that the quadriceps should always be strengthened for knee problems. It is true that in late stages of osteoarthritis of the knee, there is commonly weakness and atrophy in the quadriceps muscles. Because these muscles provide shock absorption for the knee, therapists used to think that quadriceps exercises were always in order. Recent research, however, has shown that if osteoarthritic knees are bowed or knock-kneed, aggressive quadriceps exercises should be avoided. They increase the deformation faster.

If you have osteoarthritis in your knees and they are bowed or knock-kneed, focus on the best alignment possible. Do the air squat (see page 22) using *no* weight. Focus on dropping your hips back to strengthen your buttocks. Avoid any pain. If it hurts, don't go down as far. Do not push more resistance, but focus on maintaining function.

People who have osteoarthritis and *do not* have out-bowing or knock-kneed alignment can benefit from lower extremity strengthening. In fact, several studies have shown that aggressive lower extremity strengthening greatly relieves pain and improves function in knees with significant osteoarthritis. In the past, patients with osteoarthritis in the knee were given very conservative exercises to strengthen the surrounding muscle of the thighs, hips, and buttocks and not put stress on the knee joint. It was believed that weight-bearing exercises that moved the knee joint would hasten the arthritis and aggravate the problem. But there are many exercises that you can do. The key, however, is to avoid pain in the joints, increase resistance gradually, and focus on good alignment.

Here are the ones I recommend:

1. Squats (see page 22). If squats cause pain, decrease the range of motion until your knee is pain free. Gradually increase resistance. This exercise strengthens the quadriceps, hamstrings, and buttocks. If squats cannot be tolerated, go to your local gym and try a seated leg press. This piece of equipment will allow you to use less than your body weight and control the motion better. Focus, as in the squat, on keeping your thighs in line with your feet.

2. Gluteus medius strengthener with elastic ring (see page 80). This muscle controls or prevents twisting and rotation of the knee.

3. Calf raise (see page 73).

4. Hamstring stretch with knee supported (see page 52).

5. Quadriceps stretch (see page 53).

6. Calf stretches (see pages 50 and 51).

7. Work on balance as recommended in Chapter 2 (see page 26). Damage to the cartilage affects nerves in the joint, which affect perception about joint position. This can affect balance, which needs to be maintained to prevent falls and improve joint position sense.

THE MOST COMMON ACUTE KNEE INJURIES

Because the knee naturally has some range of motion restrictions, this joint is prone to both moderate (overuse) injuries and acute (traumatic) injuries. Both types cause a tremendous amount of pain and certainly have a negative impact on your lifestyle. Acute knee injuries usually necessitate acute medical intervention—which often means surgery.

When you suffer an acute knee injury, you will know it: Often there is a "popping" sound and immediate pain and loss of function—your knee will immediately become unstable. Whenever you injure your knee acutely, seek medical attention immediately. Any symptoms of severe pain, instability, buckling, or locking of the knee indicate you may need to see an orthopedic surgeon. (This book is designed to help you deal with common aging problems and not trauma-induced ones; always see your physician for any significant injury.)

The most common acute knee injuries include a ruptured anterior cruciate ligament (ACL) and a torn meniscus.

A *RICE* REMINDER

With knee injuries, as with other joint injuries, one of the most universal (and effective) forms of treatment is RICE—rest, ice, compression, and elevation (see description on page 114). However, if you're feeling intense pain, if any swelling continues or gets worse, or if you cannot put any weight at all on the knee, you should contact a doctor or physical therapist as soon as possible for diagnosis and other treatment recommendations.

Ruptured Anterior Cruciate Ligament (ACL)

The anterior cruciate ligament (ACL) is located in the center of the knee, and is the most frequently injured ligament in the knee. It is a very common sports injury and, interestingly, is more likely to happen to women athletes than to men. This ligament may get torn when you twist or fall backward. Symptoms of a torn ACL also include swelling, bruising, and a feeling of instability. When the ACL is ruptured, the bones in the knee joint slip out of place, and this can result in further damage, especially to the menisci.

Curiously, a torn ACL is often not painful at first. Instead, the sufferer may hear a loud "pop" and experience the knee as becoming weak or "giving out."

Torn Meniscus

The meniscus (meniscal cartilage) is a spongy shock absorber that separates the thighbone and shinbone. This is the cartilage referred to when you hear "torn cartilage." There are two menisci in the knee, the medial (inner) meniscus and the lateral (outer) meniscus.

Meniscal tears often occur during participation in sports, when the knee is twisted. Degenerative changes occur in the meniscus with aging, and meniscal tears may occur as a result. The degenerative tear may occur while kneeling or without any specific incident. Usually, by the time it tears, there has already been gradual degradation from repetitive small injuries. What therapists call "daily insults" to the tissue (traumas that occur every day) can be caused by the kinds of activities I've described—misalignments in sitting, standing, and ascending or descending steps. Sometimes the person may not even recall any specific injury.

How much of this is an inherited tendency? We just don't know, but physical therapists, if they observe their patients closely, usually can find a movement impairment. If that impairment is corrected, it significantly decreases the pain.

Symptoms of a Meniscus Tear

There may be a popping sound upon injury. Frequently, there is simply a gradual onset of pain. Most people are able to walk immediately after a meniscus tear but begin limping as swelling sets in. Symptoms include pain along the inner or outer side of the knee, stiffness, swelling, and sometimes "locking" of the knee. A piece of torn cartilage may get caught between moving parts of the knee joint and limit motion or lock the joint.

Another sign: You may hear a clicking sound when moving the knee. The pain may be worse when squatting. More commonly, if you have a meniscus tear, you can't even go into a low, squatting position—that is, "sitting on your heels." The knee with a torn meniscus simply won't let you crouch down that low. (However, you may still be able to do squatting exercises as long as you stay in the painless, higher range when you're bending your knees.)

Treatment of a Torn Meniscus

The meniscus plays an important role in absorbing shock. Perhaps its *most* important role is protecting the underlying articular cartilage from wear. Strengthening the muscles that support the knee, especially the quadriceps, will help take stress off the knee joint and may also slow down the development of osteoarthritis.

The role of the gluteus medius is important because it functions to control twisting. *The enemy of all cartilage is excessive twisting motions!*

Unless you have only a small tear on the outer edge, a torn meniscus will often not heal on its own because of its lack of blood supply in its center. A meniscus tear sometimes can be repaired with sutures, but more often the damaged area of the meniscus is trimmed. The torn piece of meniscus may be surgically removed through arthroscopic surgery. As with any surgery, risks include blood clots and infection, and increased risk of osteoarthritis down the road. Full recovery after surgery takes up to 6 weeks.

If surgery is recommended, be sure to get a second opinion. The old belief was that a torn meniscus *always* needed surgical repair, but in a study published in the *New England Journal of Medicine*, researchers said that meniscal tears are increasingly normal with age in pain-free subjects. Orthopedists still vary in their opinions about whether patients should get surgery, some being more aggressive than others. But there is growing awareness that even meniscal surgery is a risk factor for later arthritis, so many surgeons are now more conservative about performing surgery on meniscal tears. I see many patients whose physician opts for physical therapy instead. They generally do very well.

ABOUT KNEE SURGERY

Surgical repair of many knee injuries is simply unavoidable, and that's okay, because it is often the right treatment. Engaging with a physical therapist before and after your surgery will guarantee the best outcome. Presurgical physical therapy will help you build strength around the injury and will help you recover more quickly. Your surgeon will prescribe postsurgical physical therapy.

The reason that knee and hip surgeries are sometimes the only treatment option is simple: Certain parts of the knee, once damaged, cannot be repaired in any other way, and if left unrepaired, you may never be able to resume the fullest range of activity possible. Also, unrepaired knee injuries (such as ruptured or torn tendons and ligaments) can lead to further injury. Repairing them can prevent damage to other areas of this vital joint and give you the fullest life and range of activities.

Still, if there is evidence of a significant tear, or symptoms such as a knee that locks, surgery may be required. During the procedure, a piece of torn cartilage is removed. (Otherwise, it gets caught between the bones, impeding normal motion.) The size and shape of the tear usually dictate whether surgery is performed. But you need to be aware of the probability that even minimally invasive surgery can put you at risk for later osteoarthritis in the joint.

From a physical therapy perspective, I am less concerned with the name of the tissue affected than I am with the movement fault that reliably replicates my patient's pain. If correcting the fault significantly decreases pain in the first session, I know the patient is likely to do well. One possible cause for increased risk for osteoarthritis after surgery is that the surgery eliminates the torn cartilage, but it does not correct impaired movements. So whether you are undergoing ACL or meniscal surgery, insist on having physical therapy afterward.

Exercises to Do If You Are Diagnosed with a Meniscal Tear

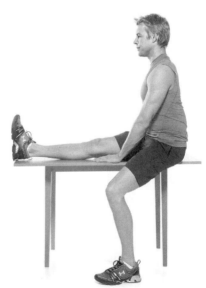

○ Do only partial squats. The farther you descend, the more pressure you put on the back of the meniscus, which is where most tears occur.

○ Avoid *all* pain. If partial squats cause pain, use a seated leg press. Move the seat back of the leg press to a point where you feel no pain when you're doing the exercise.

○ Start light and very gradually increase resistance.

○ Keep your thighs in line with your feet.

○ Do not place a ball between your knees to prevent them from dropping in. This trains you to misalign your knees without the ball, increasing twisting motions.

○ Stretch hamstrings *very* gently and always with the back of the knee supported.

- Avoid the hamstring curl. Several of the muscles used in this exercise yank on the back of the meniscus, potentially injuring it further.

- Avoid any knee pain.

- Apply an ice bag for 15 minutes after exercise and in the evening.

Pedaling for Knee Health

Many people find that bicycling, indoors on a stationary bike or outdoors, helps them recover from meniscal tears. (But never pedal backward.) Bicycling keeps your cartilage healthy. It is highly beneficial for most knee problems. Here are some guidelines when you're cycling:

- Keep the tension light to moderate and spin the pedals 70 to 90 rpms. Slower pedaling with heavy tension may provide too much force.

- Don't twist while you're on the bike! Keep your thigh in line with your foot while cycling.

- Position the seat high enough. With the pedal all the way down, your knee should have a slight bend. If you feel pain, adjust the seat to relieve any pressure that may be put on your knee.

- Try to gradually build up to at least 30 minutes 3 to 6 days a week.

THE MOST COMMON OVERUSE KNEE INJURIES

These injuries afflict people who engage in an activity repetitively and, on some level, extremely. Common overuse injuries include tendonitis, bursitis, muscle strains, iliotibial band syndrome (ITBS), and runner's knee. These injuries may develop over days, weeks, or months.

Tendons have less blood supply than muscles and so are more easily injured and take longer to heal. Resting the knee is important for recovery, and any activities that cause pain will only delay healing. Although inflammation is a part of the healing process, chronic inflammation causes progressive damage to tissues.

Tendonitis of the Knee

The quadriceps tendon hooks quad muscles (front thigh muscles) to the patella (kneecap). The patella ligament connects the patella to the shinbone. The quadriceps tendon and patella ligament actually connect to form one continuous piece of tissue wrapping over and around the patella. Both are activated by the quadriceps.

The quadriceps muscles are used to extend the leg. These tendons are commonly irritated, especially the patellar ligament, which results in inflammation of those tendons—tendonitis.

Patellar tendonitis (also called jumper's knee), which actually affects the patellar ligament, is generally caused by overuse of the quadriceps, especially from jumping types of activities such as volleyball and basketball. The pain is directly over the patellar tendon, just below the knee. Inflammation may develop. Quadriceps tendonitis is also generally caused by overuse of the quadriceps. The pain is over the quadriceps tendon, above the knee. There may be inflammation.

Knee Bursitis

A bursa is a sac containing a small amount of fluid that is located between surfaces that need to move to reduce friction. Bursitis (inflammation of a bursa) is usually caused by overuse.

The bursa in front of the kneecap (prepatellar bursa) is commonly irritated. Excessive kneeling often causes prepatellar bursitis (common in carpet layers and gardeners who spend many hours putting pressure on their knees). The symptoms are knee pain and inflammation over the kneecap and sometimes a limited range of motion. The inflammation is within the bursa, not the knee itself.

Muscle Strains

Overstretched (pulled) or torn muscles result in stiffness and pain. The main muscles supporting the knee are the quadriceps and the hamstrings. Increasing the duration and intensity of exercise or any activity too quickly often causes muscle strain. Mild muscle strains heal quickly. Hamstring strains typically occur with sprinting movements, such as chasing after a tennis ball or racing. The muscle doesn't relax fast enough as the leg swings forward.

Iliotibial Band Syndrome

The iliotibial band is a fibrous band of tissue that runs down the outer thigh, from the hip (ilium) to just below the knee, inserting into the shinbone (tibia). It helps provide stability to the outer side of the knee joint, particularly during running. It connects from a muscle, the tensor of the fascia lata, which is a powerful hip abductor on the front of the hip.

Iliotibial band syndrome (ITBS) is irritation or inflammation of the iliotibial band and causes lateral knee pain. (Despite the inflammation, you usually don't see any swelling.) This condition is most common in long-distance runners and cyclists.

Symptoms of Iliotibial Band Syndrome

Although the pain usually occurs on the outer side of the knee just above the knee joint, it may also occur over the entire iliotibial band or just below the knee, where the iliotibial band inserts into the shinbone (tibia). The pain usually sets in slowly, often after you've been running for several minutes. It is relieved by resting. But it is likely to be aggravated again by renewed activity, such as running, cycling, or walking.

Causes and Factors That Contribute to Iliotibial Band Syndrome

Overuse is usually the main problem if you have ITBS. If you increase running or cycling distance too quickly, or you don't give your body time to recover between these energetic bouts of exercise, you run the risk of irritation and inflammation of the iliotibial band. Running uphill, downhill, on a slope, on hard surfaces, or on uneven ground increases the risk of ITBS. (I see many women with this.) Another common cause is sleeping on the side with the top leg down on the bed in front of the body, which places the iliotibial band in a shortened position. Also, if you have ITBS, there's a good chance that you tend to sit with the affected leg crossed over the other.

Stiffness in the Iliotibial Band

A short, stiff iliotibial band causes excess friction over the outside of the knee—over the lower end of the thighbone—as the knee is bent and straightened. This leads to irritation and pain just above the knee joint. (A short iliotibial band may also cause patellofemoral syndrome.)

Weak Hip Abductors

The hip abductors are muscles involved in moving your leg to the side. These abductor muscles help support the knee. If you strengthen them, you'll help support the knee and often improve ITBS. A study at Stanford University found that distance runners with ITBS had weaker hip abduction strength in the affected leg compared with their unaffected leg and also compared to normal distance runners. Strengthening the gluteus medius eliminated symptoms.

HIP ABDUCTORS (OUTER THIGH) STRENGTHENING

The gluteus medius strengthener can help. When you're doing this exercise (see page 80), be sure to slightly turn your feet out to focus the work on the posterior part of the gluteus medius. Start with a lighter resistance tube, such as the green one or even the yellow. Stop if you sense pain or if you have to compensate by bending to the side at your waist. Your upper body should stay rigidly upright.

Another helpful exercise is the hip flexor stretch with a focus on the iliotibial band. You may have found in the hip flexor test (see page 42) that you encountered a bit of discomfort in your knee when that leg was hanging down. (When you turn the foot inward, it increases discomfort, and when you turn it out, the discomfort is decreased.) Address this shortness by performing that stretch frequently every day, turning the foot *in* just enough to feel a gentle stretch on the outside of the thigh and/or knee without any pain. Over time, increase the range by turning the foot in more and more as the tissue lengthens. Accompany this with gluteus medius strengthening (see page 80).

Also, alter your sleeping, sitting, and movement patterns.

There has been some controversy regarding whether you can actually affect the length of this very strong piece of connective tissue. Some physical therapists have long recommended sliding on one's affected ITB over a foam roller. This is a painful practice, and it is doubtful that pressure on one point on the tissue will increase length of the whole. (It probably feels great when you stop!) Instead, I recommend the strengthening that I describe here.

Gait Problems

Some experts believe that gait problems may increase the risk of ITBS. Wearing proper footwear will help. Shoes that show wear on the outside tend to twist the foot and knee outward, putting stress on the ITB. As soon as you detect signs of wear, purchase new shoes (following the guidelines on page 122).

Mechanical Errors

If you have bowed legs, you may have increased risk of ITBS. Bowed legs may, indeed, place undo strain on this tissue. A podiatrist or physical therapist can recommend orthotic devices or place small wedges under the outside of the feet to help decrease this pain.

Another possible cause of ITBS is limb length discrepancy (LLD), but this is subject to a lot of controversy among physical therapists. Certainly, "apparent" limb length discrepancies are very common. Real ones may not be. It takes a lot of care, training, and experience (on the part of your physical therapist) to determine whether there is an *actual* difference in the length of legs.

As part of the examination for LLD, the physical therapist will feel the top of the iliac crests to find out whether one is higher than the other. However, a difference in height can be caused by a number of factors other than a length difference in legs. X-rays may be the best way to tell whether the leg difference is apparent or real, but even these can be difficult to interpret because of errors in positioning the patient.

I use three or four different methods to determine whether someone has real LLD and rarely find evidence of it. (If I do, I refer my patient to a physician for verification.) The reason I'm so careful is that correcting for LLD, when someone doesn't actually have it, can cause more harm than good. I frequently find that patients who have had a diagnosis of LLD actually have other issues that require different treatment. For instance, apparent LLD may be due to:

○ Stiffer, stronger hip abductors on one side, which "push" the other hip higher. Some exercises to address this problem will help.

○ A lower arch in one foot. When you're tested for LLD, the practitioner needs to make sure that your feet are placed in a position called subtalar neutral (that is, with the arches positioned exactly the same). If the arch in the foot on one side is lower than the arch in the other foot, your hip may "drop" an entire centimeter. If that's the issue, it can be solved with cheap orthotics.

○ An arthritic knee that can't completely straighten. Because of the arthritis, one hip drops down, making it *appear* that one leg is shorter. (In one such case, I performed a gentle joint mobilization on the knee, and the hips returned to equal.)

That said, some people do have *real* (rather than apparent) limb length discrepancies. One cause might be a history of trauma, such as a fracture to the long bones of the thigh or lower leg. If this occurs at the "growth plates" in a young person whose bones are not fully grown, he or she may have real LLD later in life. If so, I recommend placement of a lift in the entire shoe—not a heel lift. (A lift under just the heel may rotate the affected side forward as well as elevate that side.) Lifting the entire side by putting a Spenco insole or two on the short side may be all that's needed. (Shoe corrections cannot be higher than about ⅜ inch thick or they will prevent adequate fit of the foot in the shoe.) If a higher lift is needed, I recommend that the sole of the shoe be altered by a pedorthist who specializes in altering shoes.

Because of the issues involved and the frequent misdiagnoses I have seen, I recommend that anyone who is diagnosed with LLD get a second opinion from an experienced practitioner.

Treatment of Iliotibial Band Syndrome

If the side of your thigh is painful to touch, treat pain and inflammation with RICE. Strengthen your gluteus medius with an Xering. If it is painful to perform this exercise, stop stretching the area. Sleep with pillows under your knee to keep it in an elongated, relaxed position at night.

People with a short ITB will tend to cross that leg over the other when sitting cross-legged. Be sure to avoid doing that!

Runner's Knee

Clinically known as patellofemoral syndrome, the so-called "runner's knee" is actually a condition that can affect anyone, whether or not you're a distance runner. The symptoms are diffuse pain behind or around the kneecap. The most common complaint is pain when walking down stairs. The knee may click or emit crunching noises when straightened. Some people may also find that the knee feels unstable (though usually not). Running, kneeling, climbing stairs, and sitting for long periods aggravate the symptoms.

The main cause of runner's knee seems to be what we call "poor knee tracking." The kneecap glides in a groove in the thighbone. If the kneecap is pulled to one side (that is, pulled out of its "track"), excessive friction on the back of the cartilage of the kneecap during motion causes irritation.

If you have patellofemoral syndrome, the common approach is to try and strengthen the inside muscle of the quadriceps, the vastus medialis. But trying to isolate this part of the muscle can be difficult. Recent research has shown that the leg extension exercise (often used to isolate the vastus medialis) may actually pull the kneecap out of optimal alignment even more. So avoid that exercise.

Other research has found that in typical activities, such as going up and down stairs, twisting of the entire thigh—tibiofemoral rotation—causes the kneecap to come out of the groove. So rather than the old belief that the "train is coming out of the track," the new belief is that "the track is coming off the train."

The first strategy is to determine whether your knee twists in or out with activities such as sitting, standing, and going up and down stairs. See whether you can adjust your alignment so that your thigh stays in line with your foot. It must be exact. If doing this actually does make a difference in comfort, then start changing your habits!

A common cause of "runner's knee" is overstretching of the outer hip muscles. Stop doing exercises that stretch your piriformis muscles and gluteus medius. (See page 80.) Sleep with pillows between your knees at night so that your top knee is as high as your hip. One study found that in a small number of people, a flat, flexible foot "carries" the knee in with it. In these people, a shoe for better pronation control might help. In a few cases, orthotic foot devices make a positive difference. More likely, you just need a good, supportive lace-up shoe. (See page 122).

Exercises for Runner's Knee

○ Try the squat with no resistance. If you feel pain behind the kneecap, make sure your thighs are in line with your feet, or try going only as low as comfort allows.

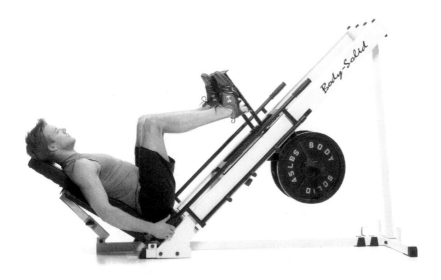

If you just can't perform this exercise, try a seated leg press machine at a local gym. This will let you use less than your body weight. Start with your knees at slightly greater than a right angle and the lightest resistance. If you experience pain, move the seat back until you are totally pain free.

○ If you have difficulty preventing your knees from dropping together, place your hands on the outsides of your knees (lower thighs). Focus on pushing out to keep your thighs parallel.

○ Do not put an exercise ball between your knees to prevent your knees from dropping in. This common strategy (unfortunately advocated in many gyms) will encourage using your inner thighs to contract. That kind of inward contraction only perpetuates the problem.

○ Perform the gluteus medius strength exercise to train these muscles to maintain good alignment!

With good prevention and maintenance, you can have knees to last a lifetime. A prime lifetime!

CHAPTER EIGHT

THE HIPS

"The history of my life is written
in my body, in my muscles. I'm very
stiff in my hips . . ."
—*Sting*

"I thought about making a
fitness movie, for folks my age,
and call it *Pumping Rust.*"
—*Michael P. Garofalo*

The history of our lives is indeed written on our bodies, and probably most of all in our hips. They're part of our "core," near the center of gravity of the body. Power movements of hitting, throwing, and jumping come from this region. We need our hips to be able to sit, stand, lie down, jump up, and run.

Maintaining and preserving our hip health is crucial to being active, especially as we round the corner into our middle years. Understanding how they're constructed and how they function is a good foundation. Once you understand the basic mechanics of the hip, you'll be able to care for them and get a lot of use from them.

ANATOMY OF THE HIP

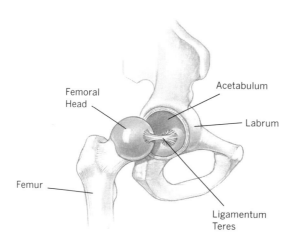

Femoral Head

Acetabulum

Labrum

Femur

Ligamentum Teres

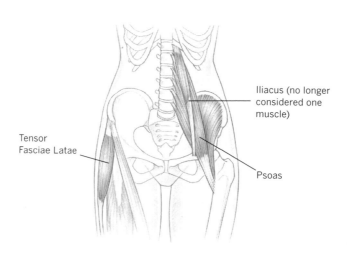

Iliacus (no longer considered one muscle)

Tensor Fasciae Latae

Psoas

The hip, which is the most stable joint in the body, has what's called a "ball and socket" joint. This is because it's capable of rotating on the head of the thighbone (the femur) at the point where it rests in the pelvic (ilium) bone socket (which is known as the acetabulum). At first glance, the hip might look like a simple joint, but it's actually quite complicated.

In order for it to function in its three-dimensional way (flexing forward, backward, and side to side, as well as being able to rotate), it needs to sustain and interact with most of our major muscle groups. It is therefore supported and nourished by a vast network of ligaments, tendons, and blood vessels. Without all of these crucial parts, the hip would not be the amazingly strong and flexible joint that it is. As we age, we need to be very mindful about maintaining the integrity of this joint in order to stay pain free and active.

Your hips need special attention to function optimally for as long as possible. To care for them, it's really important to understand how your hips are structured. Our hips are complex and multilayered. At the center of it all is the basic ball-and-socket construct, the actual joint. To keep this joint well functioning and maintain its full range of motion there is cushioning between the smooth, hard-wearing surface where the two bones (the thighbone and the pelvic bone) come together. The cushioning between these bones comes from the tough, elastic tissue, or articular cartilage, that encases the ends of bones. The cartilage, in turn, is kept well lubricated by synovial fluid. Over time, these soft and fluid tissues—with a history of microtrauma from excess stress—can wear down and diminish, which in turn causes more friction on the bones of our hip; this is when we experience aches and pains that seem to come on without warning.

HIP MAINTENANCE

The good news? There are things we can do, regardless of our age, to keep our hips supple, flexible, and pain free as we age. One of the most beneficial exercises in the fight to ward off cartilage deterioration in the hip is walking. Walking keeps the cartilage soft and promotes the production of synovial fluid, which keeps the cartilage well lubricated and nourished. (It also helps us stay in a healthy weight range, which keeps the stress load on our hips manageable.) Like all articular cartilage, the tissue does not receive bloodflow. That means the only way that nutrients get in and waste products (from injury) are expelled is when there's rhythmic movement. The movement compresses and decompresses this fluid-filled material.

Outside of the hip bones and joints is a layer of ligaments that support the joint capsule—a watertight sac that surrounds the joint. In the hip, this joint capsule is formed by a group of three strong ligaments that connect the femoral (thigh) head to the pelvis (acetabulum). These ligaments—the soft tissue structures that connect bone to bone—are the main source of stability for the hip: They hold the hip in place.

A small ligament connects the very tip of the femoral head to the pelvic socket, and this one (called the ligamentum teres) doesn't play a very big role in hip movement. But it *does* play a very big role in hip health because it has a small artery that supplies blood to the femoral head. (If this blood supply gets cut off, it can cause the femoral head to wither and die. This condition is known as avascular necrosis, and the treatment is a hip replacement.)

There is also a unique piece of fibrocartilage in the hip called the labrum that is attached around the rim of the acetabulum, the pelvic socket. The shape of this tissue and the way it is attached to the pelvic socket creates a deeper cup in which the femoral head rests. If this small rim of cartilage gets damaged, it can cause pain and a "clicking" in the hip or just a diffuse pain in the side of the hip or groin. The labrum is analogous to the meniscus in the knee. It too has more bloodflow in its periphery. There is disagreement in the medical literature regarding whether it is able to heal if torn. Some research indicates it may have a limited ability to do so.

The labrum has the important role of maintaining alignment of the head of the femur in the socket. Like the meniscus in the knee, it also helps disperse the force of body weight of the socket on the ball to protect the thin veneer of articular cartilage. Tears, the vast majority of which occur in the front of it, mean lost stability and a significant risk of osteoarthritis later. Up to 55 percent of people with hip pain have been found in studies to have labral tears. In the young, only labral tears tend to be found. In older individuals, the labral tear is frequently accompanied by cartilage degeneration, indicating that it may precede osteoarthritis.

Although not as much research has been done on the acetabular labrum as the meniscus, labral tears may be increasingly common as we age. One study found that 93 percent of cadavers had labral tears.

Damage Control

Damage can occur with trauma such as a car accident or sporting accident. The vast majority occurs gradually, over time, with constant excess stress from movement impairments. Activities correlated to labral tears include planting the foot and turning sharply away from that side, wrenching the head of the femur (the ball) forward against the front of the labrum. This can happen to young athletes, such as soccer and football players, but it may be more likely to occur when we're older and have tissues that are a little less stress tolerant. Extreme stretches that abduct and externally rotate the hip with force are particularly harmful to this structure. For example, if you have hyperextended knees and stand with your knees locked, you hyperextend the knee and hip. A hip in this position is constantly compressing the front of the labrum with the head of the femur.

In any stretches sitting on the floor, with feet together or sitting cross-legged (common stretches and positions), never try to force your knees down. There is a common misperception that this inability to get the knees down is due to "tight" inner thighs. In fact, it may more often be caused by one's genetic hip structure. Forcing your knees down in this fashion can result in an acetabular labral tear. So avoid any extreme stretches of the groin or inner thighs.

Also, whenever you're walking, focus on squeezing your buttocks together as your foot lands. You may not be able to do this all the time, consciously, but practicing it can help train the gluteus maximus to "fire" as your thigh goes back. The hamstrings, if used primarily to extend the thigh back (due to their attachment to the lower thigh and shin), tend to encourage the head of the femur to glide forward against the front of the labrum. This is one reason that long-distance running and sprinting may increase the possibility of a labral tear over time.

If you use the treadmill, it's important to be cautious. Because the action of the treadmill literally pushes your legs back, working out on a treadmill can cause you to excessively hyperextend the hip, adding stress to this vital structure. When using treadmills, focus on *not* allowing your legs to be pushed too far back. Also, limit the speed. In fact, if you have loose joints—prone to hyperextension—you might be wise to avoid the treadmill entirely. Instead, choose cycling, rowing, or swimming for cardiovascular exercise and use the Prime for Life strength routine for bone density and strength maintenance.

ACETABULAR LABRAL TEARS

There are a number of symptoms of acetabular labral tears. If you have these, I recommend that you see a physical therapist or doctor.

- Pain in the groin—or, sometimes, on the side of the hip—is one indication, especially if it is accompanied by a clicking sensation in the area. Pain occurs with lifting the knee up and swinging it outward or hyperextending it back too far behind you. If you lie on your back and lift the leg up (as in the hamstring flexibility test), you may also cause this pain.

- Certain movements or activities aggravate the pain and worsen the condition. Aggravating activities include lunges, the weight-training exercise in which you hold weights in your hands and take large steps forward, bending both knees down to a right angle. If the back leg goes much past the line of your hips, it can be injurious to the labrum. Race-walking and long-distance running can also do this. (The repetitive movement just makes it worse.) And it's decidedly harmful to perform "splits," sliding one leg forward and one back until the pelvis rests on the floor.

Here are some exercises that can help:

- Weak gluteus maximus muscles and/or psoas muscles allow excessive movement of the femoral head in the socket. It helps to strengthen them, especially the gluteus maximus. Focus on walking and squeezing your buttocks together as your heel strikes the ground. The potty squat (see page 63) also strengthens the gluteus maximus.

- Cycling can be helpful, either on an upright stationary bike or on a normal bicycle. The hip never gets pushed forward into the fragile anterior labrum.

- Avoid extreme stretching of the hip in general.

- When you're walking, don't force your feet to "toe out" if they tend to "toe in" naturally. If you try to walk toe out, this forces the head of the femur against the labrum. (By the way, if you tend to be "pigeon-toed" and naturally toe in, forgo taking up ballet. Toe-in alignment tends to come from the hip, and forcing a change can damage the hip or knees. Moms: Remember to think of your daughter with this, too!)

Tendons and Muscles

The next layer of the hip is composed of tendons and muscles. The hip is surrounded by thick muscles, including the gluteals (muscles of the buttocks and back of the hip) and the adductor muscles (on the inner thigh). The main action of the adductors is to pull the leg inward toward the other leg. The muscles that flex the hip are in the front of the hip joint. These include the iliacus and psoas muscles. The latter muscle is in the lower back and connects on the inside edge of the upper femur. Another large hip flexor is the rectus femoris, which is one of the quadriceps muscles.

The smaller muscles that extend from the pelvis to the hip add extra stability and help in rotation. The hamstring muscles run down the back of the thigh. These muscles cross the hip joint on their way to the knee and help extend the hip, pulling it backward.

Finally, there is a long tendonous band that runs alongside the femur from hip to knee called the iliotibial band. This is the connecting point for several hip muscles. Having a short or stiff iliotibial band can cause both hip and knee problems.

The Nerves

All of the nerves that travel down the thigh also pass by the hip. The main nerves are the femoral nerve in the front and the sciatic nerve in the back. These nerves carry signals from the brain to the muscles that move the hip. The nerves also carry signals back to the brain about pain, temperature, and other sensations.

When we experience hip pain, it is often due to the fact that we've either tweaked a ligament or tendon, or we've strained a muscle. Because of this, caring for these tissues is of paramount importance.

The biggest boost we can give our hips is to build and maintain strength in the network of muscles that intersect with our hip joints. Here is a look at the major muscles of our hips.

As shown, many major muscles involved in movement are attached to our pelvis. These include muscles that lead to the back and abdominal areas as well as the thighs and buttocks (the hamstrings, quadriceps, abductor and adductor, and gluteal muscles). Keeping each of these strong and adequately flexible will help maintain our hip's range of motion, which, in turn, will help us enjoy the activities we love as we age.

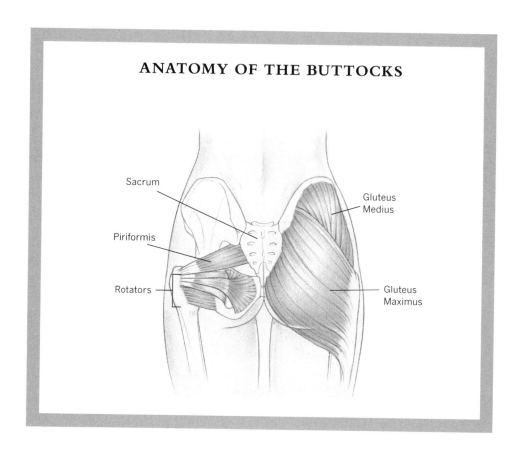

ANATOMY OF THE BUTTOCKS

Sacrum

Piriformis

Rotators

Gluteus
Medius

Gluteus
Maximus

STRENGTHENING YOUR HIPS

Hip strengthening can be easy, and it doesn't have to involve any fancy equipment. The Prime for Life strength and flexibility exercises provide complete care for your hips. If you encounter any pain with them, see a physical therapist for a movement diagnosis and ask the therapist to provide a more pertinent program for your needs. (If you have had hip surgery or have osteoporosis or any other bone or joint condition affecting the feet, ankles, knees, or hips, see your physician or physical therapist before attempting any of these exercises.)

Potty squat (see page 63): This exercise strengthens the gluteus maximus, hamstrings, and quadriceps. Concentrate on leaning forward (nose over toes) to keep the focus on the buttocks. Leaning back compresses the kneecap against the femur and can aggravate some knee problems. Always keep your thighs in line with your feet. Dropping in the knees together will aggravate your hips and knees.

Gluteus medius strength exercise (see page 80).

Hip flexion: Perform the alternative abdominal strength exercise. This works the abdominus rectus and the hip flexors. Do not add extra resistance to the feet.

Some people, especially those who are very flexible in the hip-flexor flexibility test, can easily strain the psoas muscle. Pain will typically be experienced lifting the leg on that side as you step into a car or when you're lifting the knee toward the chest. A diffuse, aching pain will often be experienced in the groin and lower back (where the muscle attaches). The best therapy for this is to avoid stretching and actively using the muscle, allowing it to quiet down. To help relieve stress, use your hands to lift the leg whenever you're climbing into a car. When the hip is pain free, start doing the alternative abdominal strength exercise to gradually recondition it. *Build up gradually and avoid all pain.*

Hip adductor strength exercise: This exercise strengthens the inner thighs. Lie down on your back and place a thick, firm pillow between your thighs. Place your feet together. Squeeze your thighs together as hard as you can and count out loud to 5 (so that you do not hold your breath). Repeat 5 to 10 times.

(Note: If you have high blood pressure or any history of heart problems, avoid this one. Isometric exercises can increase blood pressure and aggravate some heart problems. But if your health is generally good, it is another, *optional* exercise.) Remember that it strengthens the muscles of the inner thighs, but does not affect overlying fat. For that you simply need to expend more energy than you consume. Over the next year, add some muscle by walking or biking daily to get leaner.

Other Favorite Exercises to Strengthen the Hip

○ The bird dog exercise (see page 74) also trains the gluteus maximus. If you have groin pain and/or clicking, avoid doing this one.

○ Keep your hips supple by sitting cross-legged occasionally. If you are too stiff, try sitting on three to five pillows. Avoid any knee or hip pain with this.

○ The quadruped rock back (see page 48) stretches the hip extensors (gluteus maximus).

○ The hip flexor stretch (see page 54) maintains range in the hip flexors (psoas, rectus femor, and iliotibial band).

If you're experiencing hip pain, please see your doctor or a physical therapist before you begin any strength-training routine. Whenever there's pain there is a problem, and that problem needs to be addressed first and foremost. A physical therapist is more concerned about the *motion* cause of pain, rather than the *tissue* cause. Correction of movement faults is highly effective if you want to eliminate symptoms, so it's important to follow the guidelines given to you by your therapist.

(Note: Although there are many different movement impairment diagnoses, I will be discussing the most common one, hip adduction with medial rotation syndrome. Researchers at Washington University in St. Louis identified this syndrome.)

Here is a story of one of my clients at Canyon Ranch, a young woman named Liv, who knew living without pain was an option.

Liv's
STORY

Liv was a young fitness instructor who was extraordinarily fit, but she had severe, chronic pain in her right hip. Liv had seen a number of health practitioners before coming to Canyon Ranch. One physician had injected her hip with cortisone and this helped for a few days. But then the pain returned. She visited massage therapists, who said that the muscles on the outside of her hip were "too tight," and they all suggested she work to stretch her muscles, not strengthen them. (Actually, despite what her massage therapist told her, those muscles were overly flexible—not "too tight.") Someone even had her rolling on foam to stretch her iliotibial band—this caused extreme pain.

When I examined Liv, her hip joint was very tender and she had pain in both her gluteus medius and her iliotibial band. I was also struck by how weak her gluteus medius muscle was. No wonder she was experiencing so much pain!

"How do you manage your pain?" I asked her.

She demonstrated several stretches, such as lying on her back, pulling her lower leg in toward her chest with the leg perpendicular to her spine.

"How do you feel when you do those?"

"The stretches hurt, but they hurt in a good way. I feel like I need to do them."

"Liv," I asked her, "how do you sleep at night? On your back, side, or stomach?"

"I always sleep on my left side, and I kind of put my right leg across and in front of me."

Liv showed how she slept; it looked like the stretch she had just demonstrated. I asked her if she stayed in that position all night.

"I have to. It hurts too much to sleep on my right side," she said.

Liv had a narrow waist and wide hips. After I found out how she slept, and how long she stayed in that position, the problem was clear.

While I took her history, she sat with her right leg crossed over her left leg, stretching the same tissues. There was no possible way those muscles could be too short. When we tested her range of motion, she was extremely flexible on her right side. The strength of her hip abductors in the front region of the hip was strong, reflecting her regular use of the hip abductor machine in the gym. But when I tested the back of her gluteus medius muscle, which she stretched even in her sleep, it had almost no strength at all, and the strength test caused discomfort. These are symptoms of a strained muscle.

Liv's iliotibial band, the back part of the gluteus medius muscle, and the piriformis muscle were highly irritable from chronic stress—that is, too much stretching, not too little.

"No more stretching exercises," I advised Liv. "And I don't want you to do strengthening exercises either—at least not yet. I'd like to try putting tape all the way down the side of your leg to prevent further stretching. I want you to wear this all the time, even in your sleep."

Liv looked at me skeptically and laughed, but she let me apply two long strips of tape that held her right thigh slightly out and away from her body. It prevented her from being able to stretch it or do the motions that stressed it.

"Is that it?" She was obviously dubious.

"Wear that tape for a couple of days. Avoid stretching or exercising your muscles until you're pain free. Then come back."

She returned the next day, having removed the tape.

"I didn't think it was doing any good," she told me, "so I took it off." I heard her steps echo down the hall, jaunty and quick.

Two hours later, Liv was back in my office. "You know what? I think maybe the tape was helping. The pain has started to get worse."

She was leaving Canyon Ranch the next day, so I asked her to bring her husband in before they left town. I taught him how to tape her, and I gave them enough tape to last several weeks.

I got a call from her several months later, and she was bursting with good news. Liv said her hip pain was gone. She had learned how not to overstretch her hip muscles.

"At first," she said, "it was hard to sleep. The tape was strange, and I wasn't sure you were right about being overstretched. But then my hip gradually began to feel better. The tape made me aware of how often I was stretching it—while sleeping, sitting, and doing exercise."

I had given her the gluteus medius strength exercise to do after she was pain free. She had worked on it and was very strong and totally pain free in everything she did.

Liv's problem occurs frequently, I've found, especially in women who have wider hips. Sitting with the affected leg crossed over aggravates it, too. Taping is rarely needed. Stopping the stresses, sleeping with long, thick pillows between the knees, and sitting and standing with thighs in line with the feet (not allowing them to drop in) is all that's usually needed. This same movement fault also leads to tibiofemoral rotation syndrome in the knee. In fact, misalignments in the hip may be the most common cause of knee problems.

One patient who also responded dramatically to the same advice laughingly calls it "yoga butt." Indeed I have found it frequently in women who do lots of yoga with a focus on spinal twists and postures that stretch the piriformis, gluteus medius, and iliotibial band. It indicates a need for better balance in one's yoga practice—less stretching of the hips and lower back and more focus on strength, stability, and balance.

TIPS FOR MAINTAINING HEALTHY HIPS

What goes inside your body affects your hip strength. As I've mentioned previously, I especially recommend that you eat a nutritious diet with enough calcium and vitamin D (the vitamin that helps your body absorb calcium). Calcium is found in dairy products such as milk, cheese, and yogurt, and dark green, leafy vegetables, such as broccoli. And remember that if you use sunblock, which blocks vitamin D development in skin, you must make sure you get it in your diet. Follow these recommendations as well:

○ It is important to do the weight-bearing exercises that I recommended previously. Exercise and stay active. It is best to do weight-bearing exercise, such as walking, jogging, stairclimbing, dancing, or lifting weights, for 30 to 60 minutes 3 to 6 days a week. Weight-bearing exercises help build strength by working the muscles and bones against gravity. Exercises that are not weight bearing, such as swimming, are good for your general health, but do not help new bone growth. If you swim, then you have another reason to do resistance training, because it can significantly help improve bone mineral density. Talk to your health professional about an exercise program that is right for you and your healthy hips. Begin slowly, especially if you have not been active for a while.

○ Do not drink more than two alcoholic drinks a day if you are a man, or one alcoholic drink a day if you are a woman. People who drink more than this may have a greater chance of developing osteoporosis and cancer. Alcohol use also increases your chance of falling and breaking your hip.

○ Stop—or do not begin—smoking. Smoking increases your risk for developing osteoporosis. It also interferes with blood supply and healing.

○ Cut down on caffeine. Caffeine in coffee and soda leeches calcium from your body and increases your chance for developing osteoporosis in your hip and other joints.

TIPS FOR TREATING HIP PAIN AND INJURY

Hip problems may develop from overuse, bone changes due to age, tumors, infection, changes in the blood supply, or a problem that was present from birth. Oddly enough, a person who has a hip problem often feels pain in the groin, thigh, or knee instead of the hip. When you're talking to a health professional about hip pain, try to be as exact as possible in your description. That will help your health professional determine the cause of your pain.

If you are suffering from hip pain, I feel for you: There is nothing more frustrating than feeling like we're compromised to our very core. There are many types of hip pain and injury. Here are some of the more common ones.

○ Pain when resting: This pain does not increase with motion or standing. It is usually caused by a problem that's not severe, unless the pain does not go away or wakes you from sleep.

○ Pain with movement: This increases when you move your hip or leg, and the pain does not increase when you stand or bear weight. This type of pain is most often caused by a muscle injury, inflammation, or infection.

○ Pain with weight bearing: This increases when you stand or walk and may cause you to limp. This type of pain usually means you have a problem with the hip joint itself. Pain that is severe enough to prevent any weight bearing is more likely to mean a serious bone or joint problem.

WHAT'S CAUSING THE PROBLEM?

There are several conditions that can lead to hip pain and discomfort. Here are some causes of common hip issues:

○ Snapping pain on the outside of the hip (and sometimes the knee) may be caused by iliotibial band syndrome. This is a movement impairment that responds to physical therapy.

○ Pain that is worse in the morning and decreases during the day may be caused by osteoarthritis, rheumatoid arthritis, or lupus.

○ Pain may be a sign of inflammation of the large sac that separates the hipbones from the muscles and tendons of the thighs and buttocks (trochanteric bursitis). This is an indication of a movement fault most commonly caused by excess motion of tendons over the bursa. (Bursa function to enable tendons to glide over each other with minimal friction and stress.) Cortisone injections can decrease the pain of inflammation but will not address the movement impairment causing the irritation of the bursa.

○ Pain can occur with infection in a joint (septic arthritis), bursa (septic bursitis), or bone (osteomyelitis).

○ Pain and stiffening in the hip may be caused by lack of bloodflow to the hip joint (avascular necrosis). Pain in the knee may also be present. The most common cause of this in adults is a dislocation of the hip joint. It is a very strong joint held in place by a capsule of great strength and surrounding ligaments and muscles. A lot of force is required to do this, so it is rare. Avascular necrosis occurs most commonly with high-speed traumas, such as motor vehicle accidents or ski injuries.

○ Pain that shoots down the leg from the hip or lower back may be caused by an irritated or pinched nerve (sciatica) or an overstretched or irritated piriformis muscle (underneath which travels the sciatic nerve).

○ Pain with weight bearing that gradually worsens over several months may be caused by transient osteoporosis. This is more common in middle-aged men than women.

○ Some types of bone cancer (osteosarcomas) and the spread of cancer to the bone (metastatic disease) can cause bone pain.

Treatment for a hip problem depends on the location, type, and severity of the problem, as well as your age, general health, and normal everyday activities (such as work, sports, and hobbies). Treatment may include first aid measures; application of a brace, cast, harness, or traction; physical therapy; medications; or surgery.

WHAT YOU CAN DO FOR YOUR HIPS

Most problems that affect our hips are either preventable or somewhat reversible. The biggest hip ailment for those of us over 40 is osteoarthritis. Be vigilant about wanting healthy hips, and you've got a good chance of solving most problems!

PREVENTING HIP FRACTURES

Hip fractures are emotionally and financially devastating. They're also one of the top injuries that affect aging Americans. Getting into shape and staying prime for life is the *best* protection against breaking your hip (as well as any other joint or bone). Preventing this kind of fracture should be a priority for all of us.

Who Is at Risk for a Broken Hip?

Some people are more likely to fracture their hips than others, and there are a number of factors that could put you in a high-risk group. My purpose in listing some of these risks factors is not to alarm you but simply to remind you that preventive measures may be especially important for you. Here are some of the factors that are common among those in the higher-risk groups:

○ **Age.** The rate of fracture increases for people 65 and older.

○ **Gender.** Women have two to three times as many hip fractures as men.

MOVING IN SUPPORT OF A HEALTHY HIP!

● Ride a stationary bike, either an upright or a recumbent version (whichever is more comfortable). At first you may feel some stiffness, but as your joints get warm and loosen up you'll notice improved motion in your hip.

● Wear shoes that provide shock absorption and comfort. Use inserts that further cushion your step.

● The cartilage in the hip requires regular rhythmic movement— loading and unloading of your body weight—to keep producing synovial fluid, which helps keep the cartilage pliable and plump. Bicycling and swimming both provide this without applying excessive force to the hip joint.

● If you have limited range of motion in one hip, engage in gentle stretching or yoga to keep it limber. This will also help your hips stay in alignment, thereby minimizing further injury or damage. Never stretch if there is *any* pain, and always avoid extreme stretches such as splits.

● One of the most pleasurable ways to keep your hips in shape is with water exercises. When you do exercises in a swimming pool, the buoyancy of the water minimizes the load placed upon your body and, at the same time, provides resistance. Here are some activities I recommend:

  ● Ordinary swimming is excellent. If you have a kickboard, use it: You'll keep your legs in great shape, and that helps your hips. With or without the kickboard, do the flutter kick: It's gentle on your hips and most knees. You can also do the frog kick and the scissors kick if you're pain free when you do them. (As I've mentioned, the frog kick and the scissors kick aren't good for people with knee problems because they create too much twisting. But if your hips are your only problem, these kicks are fine.)

  ● Buoyancy belts let you run in the water and provide excellent results. (And they're fun!) You don't need to know how to swim to get a great workout when you're wet.

○ **Heredity.** Family history and your genetic makeup can be significant factors. Caucasians, Asians, and those who have a small-boned, slender body type are more likely to have hip fractures. Also, if your parents or grandparents have suffered from broken bones in their later years, it means you too are at increased risk.

○ **Nutrition.** A low intake of calcium, or reduced ability to absorb calcium, raises your risk. (You need adequate vitamin D—either from supplementation or sunlight—to aid in the absorption of calcium.)

○ **Personal habits.** Smoking or excessive alcohol use put you at higher risk.

○ **Physical impairments,** such as physical frailty, arthritis, poor balance and coordination, or poor eyesight, are risk factors.

○ **Mental impairments,** such as senility, dementia, or Alzheimer's disease, increase your risk.

○ **Medications.** Weakness or dizziness due to adverse side effects of medication put you at greater risk.

Prevention begins right here, and it starts with awareness. It's important to be aware of your physical limitations as well as any environmental obstacles you may face.

Five Ways to Protect Yourself from Hip Fractures

○ Exercise. Being fit and strong reduces the incidence of falls. If you do happen to fall, being strong and lean decreases the risk that you will be seriously injured or will fracture your hip.

○ Movement programs, such as tai chi (one of the Chinese martial arts, stressing slow, deliberate movements), help keep us on our feet by improving balance. Movements that require changes in weight bearing from foot to foot, along with direction changes (dancing, for instance), are probably just as effective. Keep moving those hips!

○ Increased strength leads to better mobility. Strengthen your muscles!

○ Work on increasing your bone density with a combination of diet and strength exercises. Talk to your physician and/or a dietician to determine whether supplements such as calcium and vitamin D are appropriate for you.

EXERCISE FOR AN OSTEOARTHRITIC HIP

● For existing osteoarthritis in the hip, I do not recommend using a leg press or squat for conditioning because it causes the joint to wear more quickly. Once a total joint replacement is scheduled, however, I advise patients to do both exercises (as long as there's no pain). Doing these exercises in advance of surgery is an excellent way to get in condition for a faster recovery.

● After a hip replacement, avoid doing a leg press or squat. The air squat without weight is okay to maintain strength.

● Using a stationary bike for cardiovascular exercise will help keep lower extremity muscles in good shape without excessive stress to the cartilage. After a 10-minute warmup on the bike, I recommend four to eight intervals of increasing tension (at the highest possible tension at which you can sustain the same pedaling speed), alternating with 40 to 45 seconds of easy tension at the same pedaling speed. Do this 2 to 3 nonconsecutive days per week to maintain great conditioning of the hips and thighs.

● The gluteus medius strengthening exercise maintains hip abductor strength. (See page 80.)

● The calf raise and stretches (see pages 50, 51, and 73) are also fine.

● Depending on what kind of procedure is done, it is important for you to verify with your surgeon which exercises are okay. Depending on the particular type of joint replacement, the doctor might advise against doing some of these exercises.

○ Avoid hazards in your environment such as icy sidewalks. Help prevent falls at home by removing throw rugs and clearing away things that clutter pathways inside and outside your house. Adequate lighting is also important in your home.

WHEN HIP REPLACEMENT IS THE ONLY ANSWER, GO INTO IT STRONG

When the bones of our hips become damaged and the ability to complete the tasks of daily living without pain becomes impossible, then, yes—sometimes hip surgery becomes the treatment of choice.

The good news? It doesn't always have to be a full replacement. A few years ago, a new procedure called hip resurfacing was developed. In this surgery, the femoral head is smoothed down and capped with metal, as is the inner pelvic socket. In this way, the bones are preserved. It's almost like capping a tooth. After the smoothing and capping procedure, the surfaces are able to move against one another without causing further damage or pain.

Sometimes, however, a full hip replacement is your only option. If this is where you are, being in the best possible condition prior to surgery is imperative! It is important for a successful and rapid recovery.

Worried? Don't be. Here's the story of one of my clients.

Jim's STORY

Jim was a successful local businessman. I first met Jim when he limped into my office, walking as though his right leg were hobbled in some way. It was clear that Jim had very poor range of motion in his right hip, and he was in a lot of pain.

"My orthopedist thinks I ought to have a hip replacement," he said, "but I don't want to do it. It's my lower back that's killing me."

When I examined Jim, I discovered he had very limited range of motion if he needed to use his hip in any way.

"Jim, I think it is your hip that's causing your lower back pain," I observed.

"That doesn't make sense."

"Your hip doesn't move well, and your lower back compensates with every step you take."

After we talked further, he finally agreed that, yes, his hip might be the cause of his pain.

"Why don't we try some physical therapy?" I asked. "I'd like to set a goal of restoring motion in that ailing hip of yours."

He let out a long sigh. Maybe a little bit of physical therapy would be better than the hip replacement surgery . . . I could see the wheels spinning in his head. So Jim took a seat on the recumbent bike and started to pedal. He could do that, and it boosted his morale. As soon as he was confident and motivated, we were on our way. I added other stretches and also worked on his leg manually.

Three weeks came and went. Jim was a lot stronger and a lot more confident. But his range of motion had only improved slightly. Jim knew what this meant.

He came into my office toward the end of our treatment and told me that he planned to call his orthopedic surgeon to schedule the operation. His surgeon was happy to hear that he was at Canyon Ranch and told Jim that he'd like him to keep strengthening up before the surgery. Jim extended his enrollment in the Life Enhancement Program, and I added strength training to Jim's protocol. In addition to using the stationary bike, he worked out on the seated leg press machine to strengthen his thighs and hips. (This was somewhat uncomfortable for him, but never painful.) He knew this work would help him get through the surgery. After another 2 weeks, Jim checked in to the hospital.

Six days later, I was waiting for him when he came home. I'd brought a gait belt with me to help steady him when he got out of the car. The van pulled up, and before I could offer him any help, Jim walked smoothly down the steps using a cane. He had a limp, but it was slight. We walked together to his front door.

"I feel great, Randy. You don't need to worry about me."

He had read my amazement as worry.

Jim still had some pain, but it was minimal compared to what he'd been living with before his hip surgery. His orthopedist said it was one of the fastest recoveries he'd ever seen. Jim felt that his conditioning before surgery made all the difference in the world. Two weeks later he was back at Canyon Ranch, working on being—and staying—prime for life.

The main function of our hips is to support the body while we're standing, or when we're walking, running, or involved in any activity. If our hips hurt, our ability to experience life to the max is muted. It is no way to live. Whether we use simple strengthening exercises, a combination of exercising, medication, and physical therapy, or, ultimately, surgery, caring for our hips is essential to each of us for being prime for life.

CHAPTER NINE

YOUR BACK AND NECK

"The best lightning rod for your
protection is your own spine."

—*Ralph Waldo Emerson*

In this chapter I am going to teach you how to care for your "lightning rod"—your spine. We will focus especially on the two most problematic regions, the lower back and the neck. I'll give you advice about prevention and keeping your back and neck healthy.

Did you know that almost 70 percent of us will experience an episode of back pain at least once during our lifetime? Back pain is a leading cause of disability and time lost from work in this country. The direct medical costs for lower back pain alone are estimated at $24 billion a year! Back pain occurs at any age.

As with the rest of the Prime for Life exercise program, the exercises that I recommend in this chapter are designed to be simple yet comprehensive. And some of what I say may be very different from what you've heard in the past. I want to help you take care of your back and neck—that goes without saying—but I won't be loading you up with a huge number of exercises. (There is more to life than exercises!)

In this chapter, my approach is the same as in previous chapters: I'll keep it simple. Yes, these are very important exercises, but even if you do them all daily, you'll still have plenty of time to revel in life!

HOW YOUR BACK IS BUILT

The human back is a monument of strength. Flesh, muscle, and bone are knit together in a broad expanse that stretches from the top of our buttocks to the neck and shoulder blades. The back provides support and protection for our most vital organs and houses the lightning rod of our nervous system, the spine. The intricate anatomy of the back provides support for the head and trunk of our body, strength in the trunk of our body, and a great deal of flexibility and movement. Unfortunately, despite its great strength, the back is an area that can cause debilitating pain and soreness.

Take an inside look, and you'll quickly see just how intricate it all is.

The back consists of three main parts: the neck, the upper back, and the lower back. The central feature is the spine, the vertebral column that runs from the skull to the bottom of the lumbar vertebrae. Humans are born with 33 separate vertebrae, and by the time we reach adulthood most of us have 24 due to the fusion of vertebrae during normal growth and development.

The spinal column supports our head and trunk, and it makes all movement possible. When the spine is injured, and its function is compromised, the consequences can be painful. And trying to deal with the pain and limited function is not only a major distraction, but it can also be expensive.

So let's take a moment to focus on that central support system that so often becomes a key trouble spot.

Here, in profile, is your amazing spine.

Your spine is divided into four regions: There's your neck (cervical spine), midback (thoracic spine), lower back (lumbar spine), and, at the very bottom, the sacral region, including the sacrum and the coccyx (the tailbone).

You have seven vertebrae in your neck, which are labeled (in medical terms) C1 to C7. Most adults have 12 vertebrae in the thoracic spine (T1 to T12), extending from your shoulder area to your waist. Then there are five vertebrae in your lower back (L1 to L5). Below that, your sacrum is made up of five vertebrae between the hipbones. These vertebrae are separate and distinct in children,

ANATOMY OF THE BACK

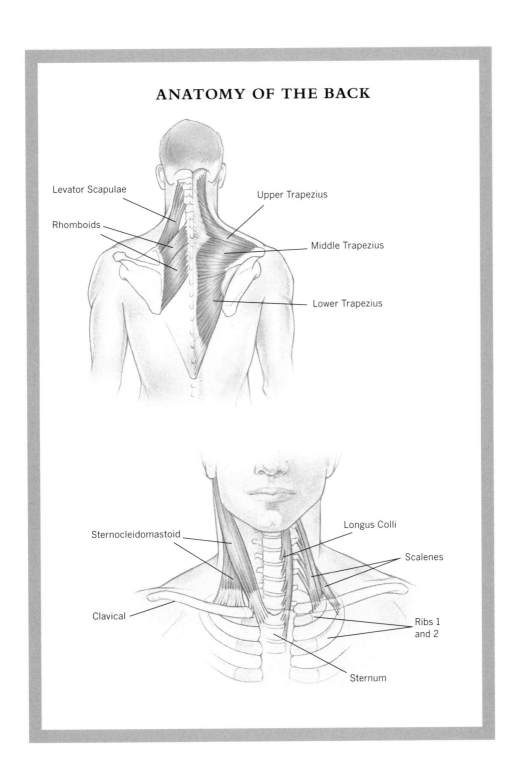

Levator Scapulae

Rhomboids

Upper Trapezius

Middle Trapezius

Lower Trapezius

Sternocleidomastoid

Longus Colli

Scalenes

Clavical

Ribs 1 and 2

Sternum

ANATOMY OF THE SPINE

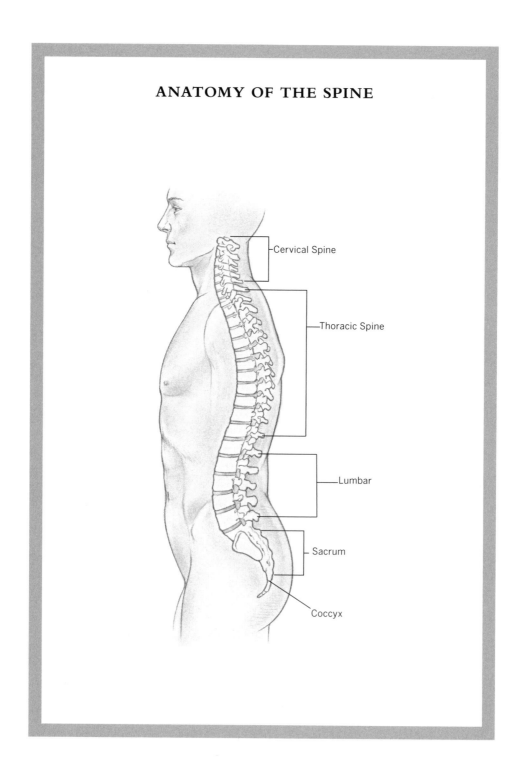

Cervical Spine

Thoracic Spine

Lumbar

Sacrum

Coccyx

but by the time you're an adult, they've fused into one bone. Last of all is the tail-bone (the coccyx), a small set of fused bones that are literally at the very tail end of your spine.

Your spine also has facet joints, which are on the posterior side (that is, the back side) of your vertebrae. While the joints have some flexibility, they also *limit* motion of the spine, preventing overstretching and injury.

Another vertebral bone structure is the pedicle. Located on either side of your vertebrae, it forms the walls of the spinal canal.

Where the Discs Are

Between your vertebrae, intervertebral discs act as spacers. Each disc is made up of a tirelike outer band called the annulus fibrosus and a gel-like inner substance called the nucleus pulposus. Although they're often described as shock absorbers, this isn't quite accurate. Discs have a high water content in the nucleus pulposus, and water doesn't compress—so they don't actually *absorb* much shock. What they do, instead, is allow bending of the spine.

Together, the vertebrae and the discs provide a protective tunnel (the spinal canal) for the spinal cord and spinal nerves. These nerves radiate to various parts of the body, where they send and receive the signals that help you feel sensation and respond with movement.

How the Spinal Column Should Look

Viewed from directly behind, the spinal column should appear perfectly straight, with no sideways (lateral) curves. Of course, the view from the side is quite different, as you can see clearly in the illustration opposite. In profile, the spine shows inward curving at the cervical and lumbar levels and an outward curving at the thoracic level. These curves permit the head to maintain its position over the pelvis, regardless of what position we take—sitting, standing, or reaching. And the spine's curvature is also an important structural asset when it comes to load bearing and shock absorption. Not only that, but these curves are also what give our backs their beauty!

Neural Elements of the Spine

The spinal cord runs from the base of the brain down through the cervical and thoracic spine (about two-thirds of the way down your back). Below about the

L2 level the spinal cord ends, and an array of nerve roots continues, looking somewhat like a horse's tail.

At each vertebral level of the spine there is a pair of nerve roots. These nerves supply particular parts of the body with sensation. If these nerves get pinched, you'll get symptoms such as tingling, numbness, or muscle weakness in the tissues to which the nerves travel.

Supporting Structures

The spinal ligaments are extremely important for connecting the vertebrae and helping keep the spine stable, especially the pair that run down the spine in front and in back. These are the anterior longitudinal ligaments and the posterior longitudinal ligaments, running from the skull all the way down to the sacrum at the base.

In addition to the ligaments, you have many muscles attached to the spine that maintain stability. The larger muscles of the trunk, such as the back muscles, waist muscles, and abdominal muscles, also provide support. In fact, recent research shows that the muscles surrounding your lower back provide an enormous amount of stability, helping protect it from damage.

The Neck: Our Cervical Spine

The neck supports the weight of our head and protects the nerves that come from the brain to the rest of the body. It is the most flexible part of the spine, enabling us to look in all directions while protecting vital structures.

Upper Back: The Thoracic Spine

The 12 vertebral bodies in the upper back make up the thoracic spine. The ribs are attached here, forming your rib cage, which is a relatively stable structure. The vertebrae on the thoracic spine provide stability and structural support while allowing very little motion. The thoracic spine is basically a strong cage, and it is designed to protect many vital organs, including our heart and lungs.

Because the upper back is not designed for much motion, injuries to the thoracic spine are rare. However, if your large back and shoulder muscles get irritated, or if the joints in that region don't function properly, upper back pain can be very uncomfortable.

Lower Back: The Lumbar Spine

The lower back, which is your lumbar spine, is capable of a lot more motion than the thoracic spine. The lumbar spine also carries all the weight of the torso. No wonder this is the area of the spine that's most frequently injured!

The motion in our lower back tends to be greatest in the segments of the vertebrae between L3 and L4 and between L4 and L5. Consequently, these two segments are the most likely to break down from wear and tear and, in later years, to develop osteoarthritis. The two lowest discs (L4-L5 and L5-S1) take the most strain and are the most likely to herniate (rupture). This can cause pain and possibly numbness that radiates through the leg and down to the foot through a very large and sensitive sciatic nerve. (Hence, the name for these symptoms—sciatica.) Almost all tissues in the lower back are capable of causing lower back pain and radiating pain down the legs.

Bottom of the Spine: The Sacral Region

Below the lumbar spine, the bone called the sacrum makes up the back part of the pelvis. This bone is shaped like a triangle that fits between the two halves of the pelvis, connecting the spine to the lower half of the body.

The sacrum is connected to part of the pelvis (the iliac bones) by the sacroiliac joints. Pain here is often called sacroiliac joint dysfunction, and is more common in women than in men. If you feel pain in this area, it might also be originating from tissues that are actually located in the lumbar spine. (This can be "referred pain," because it's essentially "referred" by nerve connections from one part of the body to another.) Muscles from the sacrum are attached to the lumbar spine, which can be overstressed, too.

The coccyx—or the tailbone—is in the sacral region at the very bottom of the spine. The kind of pain you get here, called coccydynia, is also more common in women than in men.

Physical therapists believe most lumbar spine problems are mechanical in nature. I'm going to tell you this regarding your lower back: If you feel pain there, *your pain is real!* If you have a medical diagnosis and your doctor tells you there's no reason to feel pain, *your medical diagnosis may be meaningless!* Trust your body. The pain *is* real, and it is caused by physical stresses that exceed your tissue tolerance.

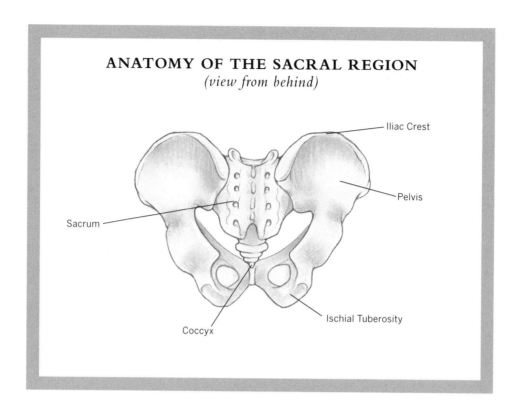

ANATOMY OF THE SACRAL REGION
(view from behind)

Iliac Crest

Pelvis

Sacrum

Ischial Tuberosity

Coccyx

DO YOU HAVE MOVEMENT IMPAIRMENT?

As a physical therapist, my perspective about spine pain is different from a physician's. Physicians are trained to diagnose problems by tissue. Physical therapists, as I've mentioned, diagnose by function. Although I have training in many types of treatment, such as osteopathic manipulation, traction, and various exercise protocols, I now use almost exclusively the movement impairment diagnostic and treatment system developed at the Physical Therapy Department of Washington University in St. Louis.

Because of recent rapid advances in physical therapy, few physicians know much about these concepts. (They have enough new literature in their own field to keep up with!) But, based upon consistent, excellent results and lots of growing research data, I have found it to be superior to other methods, plus it is gentle and safe.

Sciatica

Sciatica simply refers to pain that's felt in the buttock through the back of the thigh, to the foot (or part of the way down). This is the route of the sciatic nerve. It can be caused by many different structures—a protruding disc, stenosis, a loose vertebra slipping out of alignment, and even an overstretched muscle in the buttock (the piriformis). In treating people who have been told they have sciatica, I am more interested in what movement causes or diminishes these symptoms. I have found such symptoms to be relatively common. I've also found that the symptoms get better when people take steps to correct movement impairments.

DIAGNOSIS: A MYSTERY

When there's pain, an x-ray or MRI should find the problem, right? Unfortunately, despite dramatic improvements in clarity, there are things that can't be seen on film. And sometimes the finding isn't relevant to the cause of pain.

Studies show us that for every person over age 40 with bulging discs, herniated discs, or degeneration (arthritis) in their spines who suffer chronic back pain, the same number of people, with the same anatomical changes, don't feel any pain.

In one study of MRIs, 67 people were evaluated. Not one of them reported having lower back problems. Yet, when three neuroradiologists made diagnoses based on the MRI images, they reported that one-third of the subjects had significant abnormalities! In those under the age of 60, the radiologists reported that 20 percent had herniated discs and one person had stenosis. Looking at the images of those over age 60, radiologists said 57 percent were abnormal. Thirty-six percent, they said, had herniated discs and 21 percent had stenosis.

Other studies have shown similar results. In other words, these "abnormalities" may be quite normal. Although x-rays and MRIs may be more beneficial for younger people, the Centers for Disease Control states that "in most patients, the anatomical cause of LBP (Lowerer Back Pain) . . . cannot be determined with any degree of clinical certainty."

However, if you experience unremitting lower back pain that is inhibiting function, have severe pain down one or both legs (extending below the knee), are experiencing bladder or bowel problems (such as the urge to urinate, but inability to go), or feel loss of strength in the lower extremities, be sure to see your physician.

FINDING YOUR PATTERNS OF PAIN

A movement impairment diagnosis looks not at the tissue in pain, but at the inappropriate movement patterns that may cause the pain. When a physical therapist does this kind of diagnosis, he or she will watch you perform various movements and see whether you are doing them correctly. If certain movements consistently cause the same kind of pain, the therapist can detect a pattern. So will you!

Although this is a diagnostic process, it's actually very proactive because you begin to realize how you can turn the pain on and off by altering the way you move. Quite often, we're doing things unconsciously that irritate tissues. Once you and the therapist have discerned the movements that cause symptoms, you can begin to form an immediate plan that avoids pain and leads to healing.

Movement impairment diagnosis requires expertise, and it is beyond the scope of this book to provide self-diagnosis. The testing methods are exacting and extensive. But certain basic concepts can be helpful if you have simple spine problems. (If you have serious lower back problems, especially with unremitting pain or weakness in your legs or arms, always see a physical therapist or your physician immediately.)

There are three primary movement patterns that cause the pain. Too much repetitive movement in (1) flexion, (2) extension, or (3) rotation (twisting) will aggravate the lower back. Usually, there is a clear, pain-provoking pattern of movement, and you can usually identify *which* movement causes it. Of course, it could also be some combination of these—such as flexion and rotation, or extension and rotation.

Tammy's
STORY

I was fortunate to meet Tammy, one of the guests at Canyon Ranch, who came to me suffering from movement impairment.

Tammy was a petite, 53-year-old woman who had been experiencing lower back pain for a number of months. She'd wake up feeling fine, but as the day progressed her lower back started aching, and pain radiated into her right buttock and down the back of her thigh.

Tammy was a corporate lawyer, and when I asked her about a typical workday, she said she spent most of the day sitting behind her desk.

During examination, I asked her to move her lower back in all directions while she was standing. Everything was fine until I asked her to bend forward. When flexing forward, her spine didn't bend, and it had a slight arch. Her arching back was the confirming clue. I did the hip flexor test (see page 42). This revealed that her hip flexor muscles were extremely short. When she bent backward, she reported the familiar pain that had brought her to see me.

Although Tammy couldn't lie flat on her back without discomfort, she felt fine when her knees were bent. I tested the strength of her abdominal muscles and found they were weak.

I asked her if she usually sat on the edge of chairs. She thought a moment, and then she said, "Why, yes . . . how did you know?"

Tammy was 5 feet 3 inches tall. I explained that her height was an important clue.

"If you're short, you probably sit in an office chair that won't allow your feet to touch the floor when you're in a relaxed position. So you move forward to the edge of your chair. But sitting up straight like that, without back support, forces your hip flexors to be 'turned on' all the time just to hold you upright."

Her hip flexors never got a rest during most of her working day.

Over the years, those muscles had become too short and stiff. Because the hip flexors attach to the lower back, the overuse of those muscles made her arch her lower back (the same movement as bending backward), causing the pain that she felt.

The giveaway, in my diagnosis, was when she lay flat with her legs down. Because of her short hip flexors, she had an increased arch in her back. The front muscles of her belly were not strong enough to do their job in preventing extension (i.e., arching).

To help her correct for this, I asked Tammy to do the hip flexor stretch four to six times per day during her stay at Canyon Ranch. The alternative abdominal exercise would have used her hip-flexing muscles, so I asked her do the modified abdominal curlup (see page 78) instead. Most important, I encouraged her to select a new office chair. She needed one that would allow her to sit all the way back in the chair, with her spine getting support, while her feet were planted on the floor. I told her that she should sit back in chairs and that mild slumping, on occasion, was fine.

I also gave her the quadruped rock back exercise (see page 48), which she found enjoyable.

"It feels good," she told me.

Of course it did! It gently stretched out a lower back that hadn't done much except arch for years!

Finally, I showed her a better sleeping position. She could sleep on her back with a pillow under her knees, or on her side with pillows between her knees.

Several weeks after she left, Tammy called to tell me she had no more back pain. She could now sleep on her back without a pillow under her knees. And she had also found a new office chair. Changing her chair, she thought, had especially made a big difference!

Rachel's
STORY

When I saw Rachel at Canyon Ranch, she also had lower back complaints. Her back bothered her every day when she woke up and also when she played tennis. It was worst at the end of each workday (she was a financial advisor). As I examined Rachel and asked her to try a number of different movements, I also asked her about her lifestyle. Among the things I learned:

○ Movement testing revealed that she felt pain whenever she twisted her body from side to side. Her back also hurt whenever she arched it.

○ On the exam table, Rachel said she felt pain when she rolled over. (The movement twisted her back.)

○ Rachel told me she usually slept on her left side, clutching a pillow in her arms, with her body twisted so her belly was flat on the bed.

○ When Rachel stood and bent forward, I could see that her lower back was higher on the right. It was twisted to the right, and clearly caused some pain. Her spine looked permanently rotated in the lumbar spine—as though she had scoliosis.

○ At work, she said, her computer was on the right side of her desk and she generally twisted her upper body when she had to use the keyboard or look at the monitor.

With these discoveries, Rachel's therapy seemed clear. She needed exercise that would stiffen up her core. Her constant twisting, going as far as her spine could turn, irritated the spine in the same way that bending your finger back all day would! Her back muscles had shortened on one side and were overstretched on the other.

Rather than considering manipulation, I simply had her perform the quadruped rock back stretch (see page 48), focusing on keeping her spine straight, four to six times per day. I advised her to change her sleeping position so she either slept completely on her side or on her back—not in the twisted position she usually favored.

She had mentioned that tennis was an aggravating factor, and I pointed out that this was probably because of the trunk rotations. As her waist muscles grew stronger, I suggested this would go away, but until then, I urged her to modify her game by trying not to reach so aggressively to hit the ball. And if she still couldn't play without pain, I advised her to give up tennis until she was pain free.

Work habits also had to change. I urged her to start swiveling her entire body when she looked at her computer screen rather than twisting only her torso. She would need a chair that easily swiveled, so she could turn to face the screen head-on. Or she would have to put the monitor and keyboard directly in front of her on the desk or stand.

Rachel's symptoms were so clearly replicated during the exam that she realized, sheepishly, she had caused her own pain. By the time she left Canyon Ranch, 2 weeks later, she had already noticed a dramatic decrease in pain. Her spine was in straighter alignment as well. The improvement was accomplished by her and was much more effective in the long run than passive manipulations that I could have done. Her back problem was caused by her own movement patterns and unless she learned to change them, she would have had a recurring need to "be adjusted" or have someone attempt to "fix her."

DEALING WITH LOWER BACK PAIN

Repetitive overstressing of any lower back tissues leads to lower back problems. If you pay attention when you get the first ache or pain, you're halfway to feeling better. Most types of irritation or injury are easier to remedy with early intervention. At first, your lower back may hurt only with the specific motions that cause the problem, but if you don't address the problem at that stage, the pain can

SIX WAYS TO CHANGE HABITUAL MOVEMENTS THAT CAN CAUSE LOWER BACK PAIN

1. Try sleeping in different positions on your back with a pillow under your knees or on your side with long, thick pillows between your knees.

2. When you're in an office chair (or any straight-back chair), sit back and change positions frequently. (Your feet should be flat on the floor or supported by a footstand.) If you can't adjust your office chair to allow you to do this, find a new chair.

3. To help your spine when you're standing in one place, make sure you don't push your knees all the way back. This is especially important for people who have hyperextended knees, who tend to stand with knees in a "pushed-back" position that puts pressure on the hips and lower back at the same time.

4. If you feel pain when you arch your back, *avoid arching!* Yoga practitioners should take special note of this. Postures such as the cobra (lying on your belly and pushing up with your hands) will exacerbate lower back problems if you have short hip flexors and pain when arching back.

5. If you have a tight, stiff, rounded middle back, try the quadruped rock back exercise (see page 48). Many people with extension pain in the lower back also have tight, stiff, and rounded middle backs. If you gently stretch and straighten your spine using the quadruped rock back exercise, over time you can improve your lower back health.

6. If twisting or rotation of your lumbar spine is an uncomfortable movement, be aware, be proactive, and stop doing it!

Note: Lower back pain can be a symptom of many conditions that require medical attention, including stenosis, facet syndrome, degenerative discs, spondylolysis, and spondylolisthesis. I advise talking with your physician or physical therapist to rule out possible complications. Then make sure you *go gently* as you work to improve.

worsen. When it does, you're likely to feel pain with almost all movements. Many small stresses lead to big ones.

Whatever the issue, you'll probably need an expert to help figure it out. The pain caused by repetitive rotation of the spine—like the discomfort resulting from excessive extension—could be rooted in a number of conditions that require attention. For instance, flexion-caused lower back pain is often associated with problems such as bulging and herniated discs.

That said, here are some of the "basics" for preventing lower back pain:

○ Look at movements or positions that elicit pain. Do you sleep curled in a ball, do a lot of stretches that flex your spine, or sit slumped all day?

○ Do you like the kind of stretches that "hurt so good"? Well, reconsider. A stretch that causes pain is *not* good for you. If you feel pain anywhere—in your back, your buttocks, or down your leg—stop doing all motions that increase the intensity of pain.

○ A chair that's too low (for a tall person) can be just as problematic as a chair that's too high (for someone who's short). If the seat of your chair is lower than your knees—forcing your knees to rise higher than your hips—you'll aggravate a lower back condition.

○ If someone recommends that you should do knee-to-chest exercises, think again. The theory, with these exercises, is that you can heal your back by stretching your back. The only trouble is, these exercises can provoke symptoms rather than provide a solution. This is especially true for people who sit with their backs slumped or have to bend over a lot at work. I *don't* recommend knee-to-chest exercises.

○ If you have lower back pain, don't do the kinds of exercises or activities that force you to curl your trunk all the way forward. For instance, you shouldn't do the kinds of crunches or situps where you bend all the way forward and try to touch your knees with your elbows. Some weight-training machines or exercises force your spine forward into flexion; these are especially problematic for many people with all kinds of lower back pain.

○ When lifting, keep your back straight. *Never* lift with a rounded or twisted back.

○ Do you work sitting down? Many of us do, and right away, that puts us at high risk for back pain. The risk is even higher if there's vibration—for instance, sitting in a car or truck, spending many hours in the seat of an airplane, or operating heavy machinery.

○ Avoiding bending forward first thing in the morning has been found to significantly decrease lower back problems. Lying horizontal all night increases the hydrostatic pressure in your discs. They are subjected to a 300 percent increase in bending pressure in the morning, and the ligaments are subjected to an 80 percent increase! Avoid those early morning flexibility exercises.

THE REVOLUTION IN BACK TREATMENTS

Many physical therapists have had a great deal of success treating lower back pain. For instance, PTs have been able to treat "serious" problems such as disc bulging or ruptures (herniation) or stenosis in patients who were thought to be untreatable.

With mere movements, a PT may be able to reverse all symptoms. I see this happen all the time. Some patients who come to me have been told previously that they must get surgery or else risk serious harm (the implication being, "Don't dare do physical therapy!"). In some cases, these patients are almost symptom free in a week. But I certainly refer patients to physicians when the problem is beyond the scope of my practice.

In my experience, movement impairment diagnoses are more powerful than tissue diagnoses. If someone has a "movement fault," that subjects the tissue to stress. Over time, the repeated stress leads to pain, inflammation, injury, or damage. Microtrauma leads to macrotrauma. So, for instance, a disc may cause symptoms down the leg, and surgery may eliminate the leg pain, but unless the movement fault is corrected, the person will have recurring lower back pain.

Preventing Spine Injury

All spine injuries occur for one reason: They are the end result of excessive forces. Acute pain may come from either high-impact loads from an accident or lifting too much weight. Lower-load constant stress can eventually lead to breakdown of tissues over the years. Constant slumping, or twisting too much, can lead to disc problems. Always arching the back can lead to wear and tear of the spine (which, in turn, leads to osteoarthritis). In fact, whenever you stretch excessively, or make extreme movements in any direction, you may aggravate many lower back problems.

In the past, many experts claimed that the key to a healthy lower back was strong abdominal muscles. I believe that's only partially true. Imagine a stack of pennies on a table. If you place a tight piece of tape from the top of the stack to the table, you will have a more stable stack, but only from one direction. Add tape to the other side and you've stabilized the stack from toppling in only two directions. But if you strengthen with tape on four sides, the stack of pennies resists toppling from all directions. Your lower back responds like the pennies to the stabilizing forces of conditioned muscles. These muscles are not *just* in your abdomen. They're also in back and on both sides of your spine, radiating in every direction. The role of these muscles is to stabilize for long periods. For a healthy lower back, all those muscles do not need to be strong. They need to have endurance—the ability not to exert a lot of force, but to adequately hold for long periods of time.

Back-Stretching Exercises: An Overview

Traditional lower back rehabilitation used to include stretching exercises that would restore range of motion. Numerous studies, however, have shown that an increased range of motion may actually increase the risk of lower back pain in the future. Although we need the ability to move the lower back for function, the primary need is for stability.

The hip area is part of the "core" around which all other movements flower. A strong, stable core is less likely to be overstretched. Consequently, I do not provide many stretches for the lower back.

Some of the exercises I do recommend will "stiffen" your midsection. (By "stiffening," I don't mean that you'll end up feeling stiff and sore. In terms of biomechanics, stiffness simply means that you develop muscle strength, so it takes more force or effort to overstretch a tissue.) Your midsection can still stretch, but not to the "end range"—that is, going too far, to the point where you could damage your spine. Stiffness makes it less likely that you're going to get hurt!

To prevent back strain, you need to exercise to condition the muscles of the back, abdomen, waist, hips, and buttocks. If you leave out any one of these areas, the spine is vulnerable to damage. Research and experience tell us that strength does not provide protection for lower backs, but endurance does.

Remember, always warm up before exercise by walking briskly, riding a stationary bike, or working out on an elliptical trainer—anything that is moderately cardiovascular. Five to 10 minutes is all you need.

Back-Strengthening Exercises

Performed correctly, none of the following exercises should cause *any* back pain. Start gently. If one of these hurts at all, stop doing it and move on to another exercise. You can always try adding it later.

○ **Quadruped rock back exercise** (see page 48). This is best for individuals with lumbar extension or rotation pain. The quadruped rock back exercise gently stretches the lower back. Although it is a subtle exercise, it is powerful. (One caution, however: If you have knee pain when you're doing this exercise on the floor or an exercise pad, move to the bed. If you still feel pain, do another exercise instead.)

○ **Squat** (see pages 22 to 23). This teaches you to lift correctly. It also strengthens your hips and legs so that you don't have to use your lower back to lift. (If you have *any* existing back pain, do not use *any* resistance.) Go only as low as comfort allows. If you have extension pain, it may sometimes aggravate it. Just do a few repetitions of the squat at first and see how well you tolerate it.

○ **Practice bracing your core and breathing at the same time.** Make sure that whenever you lift something, do a squat, or challenge your lower back in any way, you "brace your core" by stiffening your midsection as though preparing for someone to punch you in the belly. Don't pull in your belly, but stiffen it by tensing. Practice doing this *with* breathing.

○ **Alternative abdominal exercise** (see page 79). If you have osteoporosis, this is the *only* back exercise you should do. The alternative abdominal exercise uses your abdominus rectus without placing too much stress on the spine. (If you have pain with arching your lower back into extension, use the modified abdominal curlup instead, and perform the hip flexor stretch.)

○ **Bird dog** (see page 74). This exercises your spinal extensor muscles, such as the multifidus, erector spinae, and buttocks. Done correctly, with *no* movement of the lumbar spine, it also activates and trains the rest of your core.

○ **Side plank** (see page 76). This powerful exercise develops endurance in four layers of muscle! The side plank helps the external and internal obliques, the transversus abdominus, and the quadratus lumborum.

○ **Gluteus medius strength exercise** (see page 80). This targets the posterior portion of the gluteus medius, which also stabilizes the pelvis. While the side plank also works the gluteus medius, the gluteus medius strength exercise focuses on the posterior region, also helping the hips and knees.

○ **All of the strength exercises using elastic bands** (see pages 67 to 72 and 80) also train your core to stabilize.

Never go to failure on any of these exercises because they can cause back spasms if you haven't built up your endurance yet. Start gently and patiently, slowly increasing your duration and repetitions.

Common Treatments for Back Pain

Bed rest used to be prescribed routinely for lower back pain, but several significant studies have shown that patients getting lots of bed rest actually did worse than those who were encouraged to keep moving as much as possible. Canadian researcher Stuart McGill, PhD, points out that when people lie down flat on their backs, it actually increases disc pressure. Higher disc pressures increase harmful forces and make your lower back more injury prone in the morning. (Avoid bending forward when you first get out of bed in the morning, and don't do knee-to-chest exercises in the morning—they are not healthy for any backs.)

For lower back pain, you want comfortable exercise rather than bed rest. Several studies have shown that walking is excellent for many people with acute lower back pain. If you experience some pain at first, try swinging your arms as you walk (from the shoulders, not the elbow). Certainly, you'll need your doctor or physical therapist's advice if you can't walk without pain. But usually it's the best kind of exercise for back conditions.

THE NECK

Do you sleep on your belly?

When you're standing up straight, does your chin jut forward?

If you're a woman, do you have large breasts?

I could go on with a similar list of questions, but by now I'm sure you're already wondering about the connections between sleeping position, chin position, and breast size. Remarkably enough, there really *is* a connection:

○ When you sleep on your belly, it forces you to rotate your neck fully to one side. This compresses your joints for hours at a time. Some rotator muscles in your neck are shortened all night long while others are overstretched.

○ If your chin juts out (from a side view, it's more forward than your forehead), you're putting constant, unwanted stress on the muscles behind your upper neck. Ouch.

○ Women with large breasts need to pay special attention to wearing supportive bras, because the extra weight puts pressure on the upper spine. Without the additional bra support, there's a good chance you'll feel neck discomfort that turns to a nagging pain.

Causes of Neck Pain

Changes in the spine in the area of the neck (i.e., the cervical spine) due to normal wear and tear are seen on neck x-rays in almost everyone over the age of 65. There is usually no pain or disability. However, several conditions do commonly cause neck pain from pressure on the spine or nerves in the neck:

○ Compression of the spinal cord

○ Pressure on a nerve root

○ Pressure from a disc

ARE YOUR NERVES INVOLVED?

Although neck pain often results from many other causes, there's a chance that it originates from some kind of nerve impairment or damage. Be sure to talk to your doctor if your neck pain also involves numbness and tingling, changes in sensation along the neck and arms, or weakness in the arms, hands, or fingers.

Evaluation of Neck Pain

When someone comes to me with neck pain, I pose many of the same questions that would be asked by any physician. My objective is to get a thorough history and do a physical examination to screen out some of the conditions that might require medication, surgery, or long-term care and monitoring. I can usually tell whether someone needs a physician who can prescribe x-rays, an MRI, or a CAT scan. Most do not.

As with the lower back, studies show that there are a similar number of people without neck pain who have the same MRI results as people who do experience neck pain. If you're experiencing pain in your neck and you have tried every conservative approach possible—this includes trying each of the recommended exercises and giving them time to work—then you might want to consider surgery. As with lower back surgery, neck surgery has an excellent track record for decreasing nerve impingement problems, but not necessarily neck pain. In some cases, your doctor might not recommend surgery.

Pain, tingling, and numbness down an arm can be caused by nerve entrapment and misbehaving muscles with "trigger points." Irritated muscles in the back, neck, and chest can all refer pain down into the arm and hand. But remember: Postural interventions are very powerful. Even the space for the spinal cord changes when your posture is altered. And when you extend your neck, the central canal of the spinal cord decreases and the cord itself is thicker. When you perform flexion, the opposite happens. As a general rule, if there is clear evidence of spinal cord impingement or fragility, it is suggested that you consider surgery. Symptoms in both upper extremities can sometimes indicate worse problems such as tumors, so if you have them, talk to your doctor to rule out such things before engaging in physical therapy. In truth, few people with neck problems require surgery. If your neck is constantly extended, it is adversely affected in a host of ways. And this is something you can learn to control!

Getting Evaluated

Although these diagnostic tools are commonly used for evaluation, they do not necessarily tell the whole story. The best care often requires a team. (I am fortunate

(continued on page 198)

Ellen's
STORY

Ellen was an active 58-year-old who came to Canyon Ranch shortly after she had been diagnosed with stenosis, the condition wherein the spaces between the vertebrae of the neck become compressed. Pain radiated down her left shoulder and to the middle of her hand. The pain would come and go, seemingly without warning. This suggested that it could be correctible. When pain is intermittent, it means that it is likely caused by a change in position or alignment.

When I examined Ellen, I could see that her upper back was rounded and that her head jutted forward. I asked Ellen to imagine, for a moment, that she was a turtle. She laughed, looked at me, and said, "I don't know exactly how to do that. Will you give me a turtle demonstration?"

"Just imagine that you're a turtle, shell and all." I said. "Now, push your face forward." She moved her chin forward. "Now, look up."

She did—and told me her pain had increased down into her hand.

"Okay," I went on, "now gently pull your head back into its shell, but without tilting your face up or down." I placed my finger lightly against her chin to help guide her as I instructed, "Pull back away from my finger."

Without changing the position of her back, shoulders, and spine (she was still "playing turtle"), Ellen withdrew her chin from my finger. She frowned and looked at me quizzically, as if to say, "Like this?" (At first it feels funny to have your head so far back.)

Yes, that was the new head position I wanted her to try.

Ellen looked at me, wondering what I was going to do next. I asked her how her hand felt. Surprised, she replied, "That pain is gone! It feels normal again!"

We repeated this sequence a few more times to convince her that when her head was forward, or she looked up, the pain in her arm consistently returned. I also gave her an explanation. When she pulled back from the "forward chin" position that she normally assumed, she elongated the back of her neck. With that, she literally opened up the nerve spaces in her vertebral column, freeing the nerves that had been getting pinched. No wonder her symptoms vanished!

Next, I asked her to lie down on her back on the exam table. "Lift your head and look down at your feet," I instructed. She tried, but when she lifted her head, she first lifted her face straight up toward the ceiling, and then struggled to look down toward her feet. (The easier way would have been simply to raise her forehead so she could look down.)

The way she moved her head, in that prone position, told me something else about her muscle strength. The deep muscles in front of her neck, the ones that flex the neck, were obviously very weak.

So here was the full story. Because Ellen kept her head forward all the time, her deep neck flexors had become too long and weak. Her neck was always extended and the top of her upper back was bent over into flexion to compensate. Until she got those neck muscles stronger, maintaining good posture would be a problem. Also, with her neck constantly extended (with her chin jutting forward), the joints and nerve spaces in the vertebrae were being compressed. Ellen had something called cervical extension syndrome.

Once I'd identified the problem, the next step was to give Ellen some exercises she could do. I demonstrated the quadruped rock back exercise and showed her how it gently stretched the rounded upper back. When she rocked back to try it, she automatically tilted her head up as she pushed back, indicating that some of her neck extensor muscles (levator scapulae) were too short and stiff.

I told Ellen to keep the back of her neck long, without dropping or lifting her head. I also had her do the deep neck flexor strengthening exercise (see page 55) and the neck stretch (see page 199) to increase her neck's ability to flex.

Ellen called back a couple of months later for a checkup. She had worked diligently on her exercises and changing her movement patterns. Ellen told me that the pain had totally disappeared.

at Canyon Ranch to have a number of wonderful physicians to whom I can refer my patients.)

A movement impairment evaluation of the neck is performed the same way as a back examination. I have a patient perform a number of motions and then report symptoms to see whether I can detect a consistent pattern. Sometimes I test reflexes, muscle strength, and sensation to determine the level of the neck involved. My interest is in replicating and abolishing symptoms, and in finding the impaired movements that make it difficult for my patient to function well and live a joyous life.

Unlike the physician, I'm not focused on the tissue, but, rather, the movement and alignment cause of the problem. Certainly, though, if the patient doesn't respond to therapy, I recommend intervention by a surgeon, neurologist, or other specialist.

In general, I believe that aggressive surgery for neck problems is risky and the results are often inconsistent. Therefore, the decision to operate depends on how severe the symptoms are and whether they are getting worse. This is the physician's decision, not mine.

Taking Care of Your Neck Pain

Here are some proven effective strategies for dealing with neck pain.

Test #1

If you have neck pain that's worse when you look up, it's likely that anyone observing you from the side would see that your chin is jutting forward. (From a side view, your ear is well forward of the middle of your shoulder.)

Ask a friend to watch and tell you what she sees as you perform the following self-tests:

1. Get on the floor and lie on your back. Gently tuck your chin in and try to lengthen the back of your neck onto the floor.
2. Now relax. Is your forehead higher than your chin? Or is your chin jutting upward with your face tilting back? If your chin is jutting forward, you have a forward head posture.

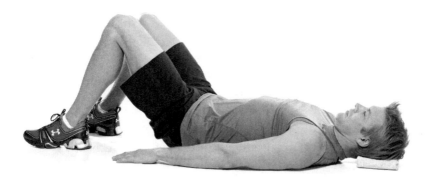

NECK STRETCH

(Note: If your neck flattens—or if you can easily get your neck down and you have pain—do not do the following stretch. You probably have cervical flexion syndrome; see page 204.)

If you can't get your forehead higher than your chin while lying down, fold a hand towel and place it under your head. That will raise your forehead higher than your chin without any effort on your part. You might have to put a couple of folds in the towel to raise your forehead to the right position.

Now, to stretch your short tissues, press the back of your neck onto the floor, elongating the back of your neck. You should feel a stretch as the back of your head slides back, *but no pain*. Hold for 5 to 10 seconds, and repeat 10 times. Do this several times every day.

Over time, as your flexibility improves, unfold the towel until your head is on the floor and your forehead is slightly higher than your chin.

CERVICAL EXTENSION SYNDROME

The cause of Ellen's pain, which is called cervical extension syndrome, is quite common. It comes from keeping your head too far forward (essentially "leading with your chin") so you have to be constantly looking up. As a result, you get what we call "muscle imbalances"—shortening and stiffening of the muscles that control the position of your head and neck. Muscle imbalances can include weak, deep neck flexors in the front of the neck; short, stiff scalenes in the sides and toward the front of the neck; and short, stiff neck extensors in the back of the neck.

To correct your head position, you must simply pull in your chin—as I instructed Ellen to do—as if you were a turtle withdrawing your head into its shell. In the "new" position, your ears should be directly over the middle of the upper arm and shoulder. The optimum position might vary an inch or so from that, but not much more.

There are a number of adjustments you can make to help correct the muscle imbalances:

- Many people, I've found, work with a computer monitor that's positioned too high. This forces you to look up. The *top* of the monitor should be about eye level and directly in front of you so that your eyes look slightly down with your face vertical.

- At night, make sure you don't sleep with one arm overhead.

- When you're getting used to the new head position, perform the "turtle exercise" with a focus on pulling the head into the shell.

- Do the neck stretch (see page 199) to strengthen the deep neck flexors.

If you continue to have pain despite making all of these adjustments, be sure to see a physician or physical therapist. Chronic adoption of this posture can ultimately lead to stenosis, disc herniation or disc degeneration, and facet syndrome. Over time, it's the movement that causes the tissue damage not vice versa.

Test #2

Ask a friend to watch you—or have a photo taken from the side—while you're standing erect. Observe whether your middle back is straight and flat or rounded.

Test #3

Again, ask a friend or partner to observe you.

1. Lie down on your back.
2. Relax your head, neck, and shoulders on the floor.
3. Now, lift your head forward as if you were trying to bend it toward your belly.
4. Ask your friend whether your face was rising up toward the ceiling.

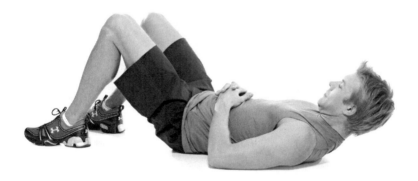

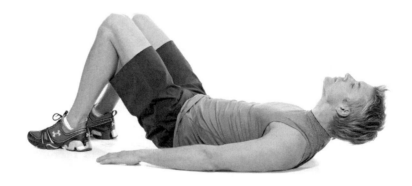

If you're lifting your face toward the ceiling rather than lifting your forehead and curving your neck, then you're using your sternocleidomastoid muscles rather than your deep neck flexors. When you don't use those deep flexors, your head is pulled forward. Large, shearing stresses are placed on your discs and facet joints. Your deep neck flexors are probably weak. The following exercise can help strengthen them.

DEEP NECK FLEXOR STRENGTH EXERCISE

The exercise is just like the previous test, but with one addition.

Place your hands under your head and literally lift it gently forward—forehead toward your navel—as high as comfort allows. Decrease the support of your hands as you focus on tucking your chin and holding the neck in place by itself.

Use as little hand support as necessary to keep the head in place. If your head tilts back slightly, provide more help with one or both hands.

As you become stronger, decrease use of the hands until you can bend the head up by itself with no hands. (Make sure, when you're giving your head this assist, that you bend it forward; don't lift your head straight up toward the ceiling.)

STRETCHES FOR THE MIDDLE BACK

If you have a rounded spine, a forward-jutting head, and a history of neck pain, you will need to do some stretches for the middle back. Perform the following tests and stretches:

- The latissimus dorsi test (see page 39)
- The "L" stretch (see page 47)
- The quadruped rock back stretch (see page 48)

As you do these stretches, focus on keeping your neck in line with your spine.

Test #4

1. Stand up.

2. Push your shoulders down as far as you can. Imagine that you're holding something heavy in each hand.

3. Keeping your shoulders down, turn your face as far as you can to the right.

4. Repeat, turning your face as far as you can to the left.

5. Now, sit in a chair with high armrests. (The armrests should be high enough to bring your shoulders up level with the base of your neck—parallel with the floor—when your forearms are flat on the armrests. If you need additional height, just add some rolled-up towels to the tops of the armrests.)

6. Relax your elbows and let your shoulders down.

7. Turn your face to the right as far as you can.

8. Repeat, turning your face to the left.

Now for a quick analysis. Was it more difficult to turn your head when your shoulders were down? Did it become easier when your elbows were supported? Which shoulder position was more comfortable for your neck?

Correction for Sloping Shoulders

Notice that when your shoulders are supported and up (relaxed, not tensed) you have a greater range of motion and comfort level. For individuals whose shoulders slope downward, the simple act of support can make an enormous difference. When your shoulders push down, there's a lot of force on the discs and facet joints. The downward force on the neck can actually contribute to problems such as disc herniations, arthritis, and even chronic headaches. When sitting, always make sure that your arms are supported on armrests at the correct height, so you can maintain level shoulders without a lot of effort. When standing, it helps to place your hands on your hips to help level your shoulders into a more relaxed position and relieve some of the downward pressure.

The Connection between Your Neck and Headaches

We've known about the connection between the neck and headaches for a long time. One kind of headache in particular—where you feel pain in the eye region—is commonly caused by the compression of a nerve that lies between several upper vertebrae. If you do get headaches, there's a good chance that a change of shoulder position can help alleviate the problem.

Allowing your shoulders to be up (but not tensed up) and giving them support when needed can maintain or create a healthy neck. This can allow a strained neck to heal faster, too. And if you've been coping with headaches, maybe they'll go away.

Here are things you can do to take tensile loads off the neck and decrease stress:

○ Keep your shoulders passively elevated to maintain level shoulders.

○ Raise the armrests on your desk chair.

○ When you're sitting at a table, put your elbows on the table.

○ When standing, fold your arms across your chest, place your hands on your hips, or (if you're wearing a jacket) place your hands in your jacket pockets.

○ Avoid carrying a heavy bag with the strap over one shoulder. Do not stretch the neck sideways and/or press either shoulder down, because overstretching the upper trapezius muscle will worsen this problem. Heavy bags do the same thing as the stretch. Avoid both.

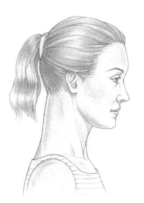

Correcting for Cervical Flexion Syndrome

If you experience pain when you look down, you may have cervical flexion syndrome. As shown in the illustration, there is a decrease in the inward curve of the neck.

Sometimes the syndrome is caused—

MAINTAIN PROPER POSTURE . . .
EVEN WHILE YOU'RE SLEEPING!

It is important that you have proper support at night when you're in bed. A good mattress will conform to your spine's natural curves and keep your spine in proper alignment. If it's too firm or too soft, your mattress can cause problems.

Even with the right mattress, though, you can aggravate back-related problems if you have the wrong sleeping posture. Here are some guidelines:

- If lying on your back causes neck pain, it may be caused by having a pillow that's too high. Sleeping in this position, you should have a pillow just thick enough to keep the neck in a straight line with your spine.

- If you normally lie on your stomach, change position to lie on your side. Lying on your stomach increases the curve of your lower back, leads to shortening of the muscles in your lower back, and encourages swayback. When you *just* turn your head to the side, it can shorten your neck muscles and compress the facet joints on one side, leading to disc problems and stenosis. You need to be fully on your side, so there's no twisting of your spine or neck at night.

- On your side, the best position is with your knees bent and a large, thick, long pillow between your knees. This sleeping position prevents overstretching the piriformis muscle, which is a common cause of sciatic symptoms. The pillow should be long enough that your top leg can't easily fall off and down onto the bed. "Body pillows" are usually about 6 feet long and are excellent for this.

ironically enough—by focusing on "good posture." If you stand or sit in an *overly* erect manner, your shoulders may fall too low, which accentuates the lengthening of your neck. (To see this in its most exaggerated form, you can look at the posture assumed by highly trained ballet dancers who *want* to accentuate the length of their necks.)

There are also a number of unconscious ways you may be forcing your neck to flex too much. For instance, you should avoid reading in bed with a pile of pillows under your head. In that position your neck flexes too much because it is bent forward too much. Shoulders that are too low are an accompanying postural fault that also pulls down on the neck, adding to the problem.

To help correct your neck position and avoid cervical flexion syndrome:

○ When seated at a desk and reading, use a book holder to avoid looking down.

○ When resting or sleeping on your back, place a small rolled-up towel under the neck.

○ Look up frequently.

○ If your shoulders are downward sloping, sit in a chair that has high armrests (or make the adjustments described earlier) so your shoulders level out when your forearms are resting on the armrests.

BACK AND NECK HEALTH TIPS

With a healthy back, you'll be able to participate in the activities you love, and even try out some new moves. Dancing, jumping, swimming, making love, hiking, rafting, playing tennis . . . a healthy back is important in keeping you fit and prime for all these activities.

Regular exercise is one important key to maintaining a healthy back, but be sure to avoid any activities that cause back or neck pain. In addition:

○ Maintain good posture, and give your back the support it needs.

○ Invest in a good pillow and mattress.

○ Invest in the right desk and chairs.

○ Remember that there is no ideal sitting posture. It is fine to slump as long as you also sit up straight sometimes, tilt the chair back, etc. Stand up at least once every hour—or more. Change positions frequently!

○ Always attempt to carry items heavier than 10 pounds in a balanced fashion, dispersing the weight as evenly as possible from right to left. Don't overload your luggage, backpack, or purse.

○ Use proper phone technique and equipment. Don't cradle your phone between your neck and shoulder. Use a headset to keep your head in a neutral position if you're going to talk for a long time.

○ Don't smoke. Smoking increases the risk for many life-threatening conditions and others that are more benign—this includes lower back pain.

○ If you're a woman, wear a good, supportive bra. Get properly fitted and wear a bra that fits your body—this will reduce neck, shoulder, and back strain.

○ Increase your core strength. Having strong "core" muscles helps support your lower back and pelvis. By strengthening your core muscles, you'll increase spinal stability and reduce back pain.

○ Adjust your posture frequently. Alternate between sitting and standing tasks to reduce the stress placed upon the spine, your back, and neck.

CHAPTER TEN

THE SHOULDERS

Choose a subject equal to your abilities;
think carefully what your shoulders
may refuse, and what they are capable of
bearing.

—Horace

When you feel as if the weight of the world has settled on your shoulders, imagine an angel whispering in your ear, "Go easy on yourself. Unburden. Relax. . . ."

Easier said than done, right? Especially in a world where our shoulders are involved in so many activities that stress them—peering at a computer screen for hours a day, reaching high to grab something off the top shelf, toting bags of groceries into the house. Tension rides on our shoulders as we move through our hectic lives.

So . . . angelic intervention might sound great, but where is it when it comes to the heavy lifting of daily life?

In fact, you are your own best counselor. You just need to learn how to move through this world in comfort. In this chapter, I'll coach you in practical ways to achieve pain-free shoulders. (Not surprisingly, some of this advice is close to, or

NOTHING SHOULD HURT

Severe pain in the shoulder can be caused by things that are surprising. Gallbladder problems often send "referred" pain to the right shoulder. (In other words, there may be something seriously wrong with your gallbladder, but where you *feel* the pain is in the shoulder rather than in your gut.)

Certain tumors can occur in the shoulder area. Left shoulder, neck, jaw, or arm pain can be indicative of heart problems. Sometimes women's reproductive system problems can refer pain to the shoulders, too.

If pain increases with anything we do in this chapter, discontinue and see a physical therapist or your physician. *Nothing should hurt at all.*

the same as, my prescriptions for a pain-free back and neck.) I think you'll be amazed when you see how small changes can make a huge difference. But the *daily* self-training for what your shoulders need is up to you. Again, being proactive makes you feel good. We have the right and responsibility to be in charge of our own bodies!

That said, if I were your angel, here are some of the things I would whisper in your ear, from time to time, as gentle reminders:

○ Maintain good shoulder posture.

○ When you lift your arms over your head, let your shoulders rise up naturally.

○ If you have to sit for long periods of time, find a chair with armrests and adjust them to the proper height.

○ Avoid wrenching or twisting your shoulders by lifting anything that's too heavy.

○ When you feel shoulder pain, stop what you're doing.

○ If the pain continues, don't resume your sport or activity until you've had a chance to meet with a health professional for a diagnosis.

These pieces of advice will mean more to you as you read on. For instance, it takes some knowledge of shoulder structure to understand what's meant by "good shoulder posture." And as I've suggested, there are shoulder injuries that can't be repaired by changing your habits, so I'll discuss them, too. But if you feel right now as though you're bearing the weight of the world on your shoulders, maybe I can help lift some of that.

WORKING WITH SHOULDERS

As a physical therapist, I frequently see clients diagnosed with rotator cuff tears, impingements, or bursitis. When they reach up, their shoulders hurt. The activities that they used to love, such as tennis or swimming, become excruciating. Occupations that require them to raise their arms above their shoulders or above their heads become difficult or impossible.

Although there are many causes of shoulder pain, the types described here are the most common. Understanding a little about them can help you prevent or treat some simple but painful problems.

A Joint Venture

First I'll share what I know with absolute certainty about our shoulders: Each is an extraordinary system of four joints and many muscles that enable us to hit tennis balls and home runs, to swim, and to dance while we shake our arms with wild abandon above our heads. Our shoulders allow us to exert tremendous force, yet they control the dexterous and delicate movement of our hands. This complex system makes our species unique.

And things do go wrong.

Iris's
STORY

Several years ago I saw a young woman named Iris who was in her mid-thirties and complained of shoulder pain. Iris was trim and fit, but it was becoming difficult for her to reach her arms above her shoulders. As a matter of fact, many of her daily activities were becoming painful.

The examination began. She showed typical signs of impingement. While I gently pushed her humerus (the top of the arm bone) up against her acromium (the place that the shoulder blade attaches to the collarbone), she said she felt a sharp pain on top of her right shoulder. This test compresses the rotator cuff between the underside of the shoulder blade and humerus, pinching them. Pain indicated there was a probable impingement of the rotator cuff muscle.

Using some standard physical therapy tests, I checked the strength of her rotator cuff muscles. They were strong. Her posture looked good. Her spinal alignment was excellent, but her shoulders were too low. (Although all shoulders slope slightly down from the neck and out, hers did so at a significantly severe angle.)

I asked Iris to reach up. She didn't elevate her shoulders at all, and she felt pain. Looking at her shoulder blades as she did this, it was easy to see that they didn't rotate up enough. I helped her by putting my hands under her armpits and lifting them as she reached up. Iris reported no pain. None!

Now a treatment plan was in view. When her shoulders were supported and moved up with her arms, she had no pain because the pinching of her rotator cuff muscles was stopped!

Next, I asked her to shrug her shoulders—that is, lift them upward—as she also reached her arms overhead. She said she'd been taught never to do that.

"Humor me," I said.

She did. She admitted that her pain decreased quite a bit. With further muscle testing we discovered which muscles were too short and stiff.

One thing causing Iris's pain was her dancer's shoulder posture. In their training, dancers are told to keep their shoulders down. It accentuates the line and length of the neck, and is one reason that ballet dancers acquire long, slender necks. That might be good for ballet. In order to do that, they have to overstretch the upper trapezius muscle. That drops the shoulder blades down but also causes problems.

In order to reach up, normal shoulder blades must rotate out and up enough to prevent pinching of the rotator cuff muscles. Iris needed to learn to allow her shoulders to rise up naturally whenever she reached up.

I gave her exercises to do four or more times each day. Our goal was to train her to shrug up, using her upward rotating muscles, and to stretch her short, stiff muscles. She had an excellent prognosis.

I saw Iris about a week later and asked about her shoulder.

"Oh," she said. "I found a massage therapist who worked on me. She said the top of my shoulder was in a spasm. It feels much better now."

For Iris's sake, I was glad that she'd found treatment for the pain. But privately, I wondered whether massage was really going to address the mechanics of her shoulder problem. Sure enough, when I saw her again in the resort several weeks later, Iris told me her shoulder still hurt.

I wasn't surprised. Despite the fact that her shoulder pain was easily diagnosed, and her treatment outcome looked good, her problem wasn't going to go away with massage treatments. I knew Iris would have to unlearn what she had created and took great pride in—her beautiful upper-body carriage. It was just too difficult for her to believe that years of training in dance could be hurtful.

Just as in other therapies, successful physical therapy requires more than the effort of simple exercises. We must commit to changing who we are. Sometimes we must leave the comfort of a familiar self-image in order to change and live without pain. All musculoskeletal pain boils down to this—retraining your brain.

HOW YOUR SHOULDER WORKS

To understand how to keep your shoulders prime for life, it's helpful to understand the basics of the anatomy.

A Close Look at the Rotator Cuff

The main shoulder joint, the glenohumeral, is a ball and socket joint. The round head of the humerus (your upper arm) fits into the concave part of your scapula. In this area the stability of your shoulder is maintained by four muscles—the supraspinatus, infraspinatus, teres minor, and subscapularis. These muscles make up your rotator cuff.

The Rotator Cuff Muscles

The rotator cuff muscles keep the head of your humerus seated in the socket. Without your rotator cuff your larger, stronger muscles—such as the latissimus dorsi in your back and the pectoralis major in your chest—could slide off the top of your arm bone in various directions, damaging your joints, cartilage, and other bones.

As we age, many of us experience pain because we injure our rotator cuff. (Iris was fortunate. Being young, she probably just had an irritated or inflamed rotator cuff tendon or irritation of the fluid-filled sac that cushions the tendons.) When the rotator cuff is injured, sharp pain shoots along the top of the shoulder. The pain may radiate down the side or front of the shoulder.

But, over time, chronically irritated tissues become more vulnerable to damage.

The Fulcrum for Your Shoulder Joint

Your shoulder area also includes the sternoclavicular joint. This is the interface between your breastbone (sternum) and your collarbone (clavicle). To feel this joint, place your left hand on your right sternoclavicular joint (SC joint), shown in the illustration on the opposite page, and swing your right arm up and over your head.

You'll feel the movement beginning at this joint. It is the fulcrum for your entire shoulder joint. The clavicle swings from this point, carrying up your entire shoulder.

ANATOMY OF THE SHOULDER

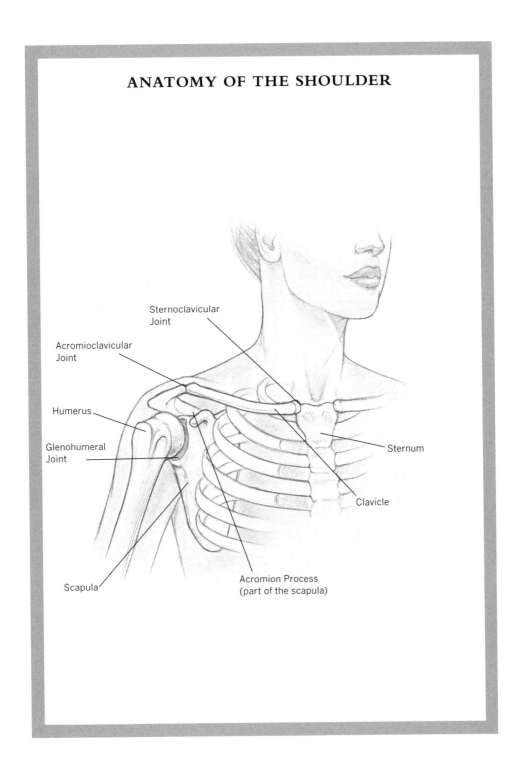

Sternoclavicular Joint

Acromioclavicular Joint

Humerus

Glenohumeral Joint

Sternum

Clavicle

Scapula

Acromion Process
(part of the scapula)

ANATOMY OF THE SHOULDER MUSCLES

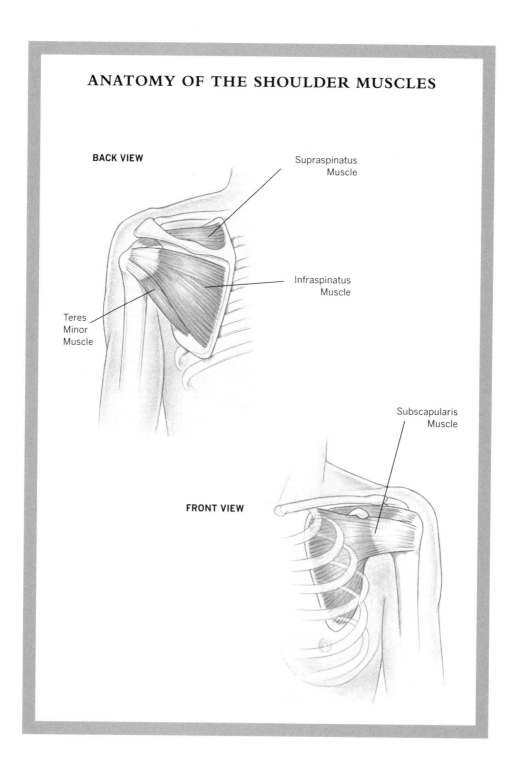

BACK VIEW

Supraspinatus
Muscle

Infraspinatus
Muscle

Teres
Minor
Muscle

Subscapularis
Muscle

FRONT VIEW

The Acromioclavicular Joint

At the other end of the collarbone is the acromioclavicular (AC) joint. The seat of this joint, the acromion, is the bony end of your scapula or shoulder blade. You can feel it on the outside and top of your shoulder. The AC joint is somewhat rigid, and it's held together firmly with tough ligaments like the other tough connective tissues that hold bone to bone throughout your body.

Sometimes abnormal muscle control causes stress to this joint. With reaching motions it may click. Although not necessarily painful, this can sometimes indicate a potential problem area.

The Glenohumeral Joint

Just below is the glenohumeral joint (GHJ), the ball and socket joint. From that joint your arm pivots with greater mobility than any other joint in your body. The GHJ requires the strength of the surrounding muscles to work correctly. All movements of the GHJ are accompanied by the contraction of the rotator cuff muscles.

The Scapulothoracic Joint

The final joint in the shoulder area is called the scapulothoracic "joint" even though it isn't a real joint. It's the interface where the muscles surrounding your mobile shoulder blade meet up against your rib cage. The scapula glides against the rib cage in multiple directions to accompany the movements of the GHJ. It provides enough stability to allow an enormous range of motion. That range lets us do things that are as different as pushups, pullups, lifting children, and casting a fishing line.

Impingement, bursitis, tendonosis, rotator cuff tear, and osteoarthritis—all can be caused by too much pressure on the tissues directly below the acromion (called the subacromial space). Most commonly, this space diminishes over time because the muscles that prevent the upward rotation of your shoulder blades become too short and stiff. With the loss of a few millimeters of space, you're likely to start getting painful shoulders.

The muscles between your shoulder blades, the rhomboids, pull your shoulder blades together and rotate them down. If you overwork the rhomboids with exercises such as rowing, they can shorten and resist upward rotation. That's when impingement occurs. The same thing can happen if you have large, heavy shoulders or if you overstretch your upper trapezius along the upper shoulders

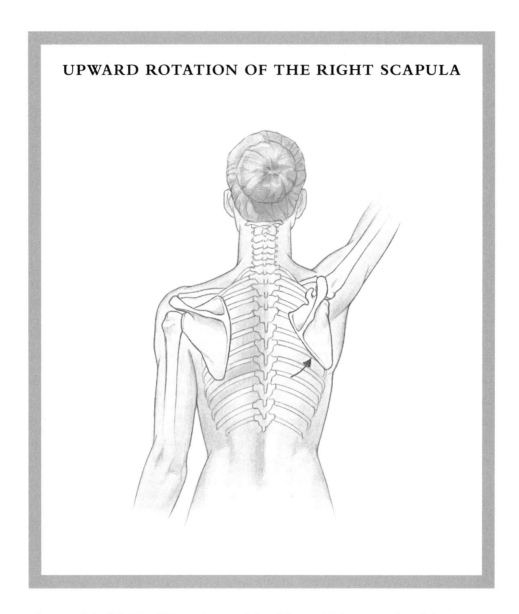

UPWARD ROTATION OF THE RIGHT SCAPULA

(the way Iris did). You'll have lowered shoulders, which means there's inadequate room, underneath, for shoulder motion.

Shoulder disorders are characterized by a dull, aching pain on the front and outside of your upper arm, sometimes radiating to your elbow. Other signs? If you sleep with your weight on your shoulder, it may be painful in the morning. And, when raising your arm up from your side, you may feel a sharp, stabbing pain.

WHY IT HURTS SOMETIMES

Shoulder pain, soreness, or arm pain may be traced to a number of causes. Among them:

- Impingement: When there is not enough space between the humerus (upper arm bone) and the acromium, it's called impingement. Tissues that become trapped in this space include the rotator cuff and the bursa. Pressure against the underside of the acromium may cause bony "spurring"—that is, a growth of extra bone, creating a "spur" that interferes with movement.

- Tendonitis or tendonosis: This occurs when the connective tissue that attaches muscle to bone is either irritated and inflamed (tendonitis) or degenerating from chronic overstress (tendonosis).

- Rotator cuff tear: Torn rotator muscles are diagnosed by an MRI. (Your doctor or physical therapist can perform simple tests that usually indicate whether an MRI is even necessary.) Mild tears may respond well and heal with therapy. A full-thickness, complete tear requires surgery so you can return to the activities you love.

- Bursitis: An inflammation of the bursa, the protective fluid-filled sac around the joint, can cause pain with all movements, passive and active. Doctors will often recommend injections of corticosteroids to decrease inflammation, but unfortunately this medication also decreases the strength of connective tissue. Many physicians believe that two or three injections in a 2-year period is the safe, maximum dose. (But, in any case, shots do not address the biomechanical problem.)

- Osteoarthritis: This is the condition I've described earlier, a degeneration of the pearly white, slippery substance—your cartilage—that lines all major joints. When it's gone, the body tries to compensate by building up extra bone. But bone doesn't provide the necessary "glide and slide," nor does it absorb shock the same way cartilage does. The friction of bone against bone causes osteoarthritis.

LOOKING FOR CAUSES

Common medical diagnoses typically target the source of the pain, but not the cause of the problem. Consequently, if you have surgery to remove a bone spur, that might help relieve stress on the tissues, and the pain could decrease or be eliminated. That's the good news. But the *cause* of the problem is not just the spur that reduces space. It's also excess stress on connective tissue and muscles.

So a physical therapist will take a different approach, attempting to find out whether there's some decreased upward rotation of the scapulae with elevation of the upper arm or other muscle imbalances that prevent adequate clearance of the humerus under the acromion. Impingement, bursitis, and stress to the bone and rotator cuff tendons are often simply manifestations of the scapula not swinging up enough.

While the source of the pain is the impinged tissue, the real cause may be the restriction of the scapula or humerus, which are the powerful muscles of your back or chest. A physical therapist can examine your arm motion and find out. But even though you may need a physical therapist to determine *exactly* which tissues aren't working properly, many people can avoid problems in the first place with the right kinds of exercises. The exercises in this chapter will painlessly help many people who have early signs of shoulder problems, but remember that there are many movement impairments of the shoulder that can lead to identical problems.

Sam's
STORY

Sam had more shoulder misery than Iris (the dancer), and he had the same diagnosis. Despite being twice her age, Sam decided to change. And he did.

For a couple of years, Sam had been complaining about having pain in both of his shoulders. He tried to ignore the pain at first, but decided to seek out a professional when it got to the point where he could barely lift his arms as high as his shoulders without excruciating pain in both shoulders. I offered to help, but Sam didn't seem to think a few exercises could do very much. His doctor referred him to an orthopedic surgeon.

Sam saw the surgeon, had x-rays and an MRI, and learned he had rotator cuff tears and bony spurs in the space between his shoulder blade and the humerus. Sam was told he needed surgery, a "subacromial decompression," to remove the spurring and mend the partial tear in his rotator cuff. (You can imagine how thrilled he was to receive that news!) Both arms needed to be done, but because there is risk with any surgery, the doctor suggested that Sam get a surgical repair of his right shoulder first. If that operation went well, the other shoulder could be repaired the following year.

As the time of surgery drew near, Sam became excited . . . in a positive way. (This alone shows his level of pain and desperation. Surgery is something people are rarely excited about, especially when the word *risk* is figured in.) This usually stoic man was suffering terribly. It had gotten to the point where he winced any time he reached up with either hand. June came, and so did the surgery. We all rooted for Sam and a new life without pain.

Several weeks passed. When I next spoke to Sam, it was after his surgery, and there was disappointment in his voice when he told me his pain relief was only marginal. I reassured him, saying healing takes time, and suggested that in a few months his shoulder would probably feel as good as new. Indeed, after 3 months with some physical therapy, he was happy with the results. He became, at last, pain free.

Then he started obsessing about his left shoulder. It still hurt a lot.

With several months left before the next surgery, Sam came to me and asked if I could help decrease the pain a bit until his next surgery.

"I'll try anything," he said. "I don't know how much longer I can keep going on this way."

In evaluating him, I noticed a crease in the skin between his shoulder blades. "Do you work on keeping your shoulders back?" I asked him.

"Yes," he answered with pride. "I learned good posture in the Navy and I haven't forgotten it."

Habitually squeezing your shoulder blades together, overworking the rhomboid muscles, can greatly limit normal shoulder blade motion and lead to shoulder problems. Judging by the visible crease in his skin and Sam's own definition of "good posture," I guessed he'd been over-working those muscles for years.

Sam's shoulder blades were about an inch and a half from his spine. Three inches is normal, no matter what size the person is. As I examined and tested the muscles around Sam's shoulder, I could ascertain that the head of Sam's left humerus was being pushed forward in its socket. His pectoralis major muscle and latissimus dorsi muscles were too short and stiff, which meant they interfered with normal, upward rotation.

When I looked at Sam's surgically repaired right arm, I had further bad news. Though Sam reported himself pain free for the moment, there were signs that this wouldn't last long. In fact, his right arm had more serious faults than the left. The surgical fix had provided more space for the tissues between the scapula and the humerus, but the cause of the problem had not been addressed. While Sam's surgery had bought him time, I guessed the problem in his shoulder might return. (Of course, that's not what you want to hear if you've just gone through one surgery and another is around the corner!)

After determining the cause versus the source of his pain, we went to work creating a permanent solution. I gave Sam new exercises that would stretch his short, stiff muscles, including the quadruped rock back as well as the latissimus dorsi and chest stretches. Sam stretched for 30 seconds four to six times each day. His muscles, which should have been upwardly rotating his shoulder blades, were on permanent vacation.

He had to be cautioned not to go to pain.

"I thought it was 'no pain, no gain,'" he said.

"Sam," I replied, "that expression—'no pain, no gain'—it means 'no brain!'"

He laughed, but the point was made. It was important for him to realize that when he had pain, it meant he was exceeding tissue tolerance. I wanted him to start feeling good again when he was exercising.

Another thing I discovered during my exam was that Sam's shoulder sloped down too much from his neck to his shoulders. So did his collarbones. This meant that when he reached up, his shoulder blades were starting from a position that was too low. I urged him to use high armrests when he was seated at his job.

At first, I helped show him the right way to lift his arms, so he would get in the habit of doing so, even when I wasn't there to help him. I trained him to allow his shoulders to naturally rise when reaching up.

Sam was a big project. Not for me, but for himself. On the other hand, he was working for a long-term solution and he was being what he's been his whole life—proactive.

Sam's left shoulder started to improve. After 2 months he said his pain was nearly gone. Three months later he said that he'd suddenly realized he hadn't felt any pain for a while. He cancelled the scheduled surgery and had one more story under his belt about beating the system.

A NOTE FOR DANCERS AND STUDENTS OF PILATES

Individuals with a dance background or Pilates training are often taught to press their shoulder blades down while elevating their arms.

It's poor body mechanics.

Although you may need to keep your shoulders down while you dance or practice Pilates, I don't advise you to maintain that posture when you're outside the studio. Follow the guidelines for normal shoulder posture whenever you're not on the dance floor. Always honor the proper alignment of your shoulder by reaching out or up at an angle that is slightly forward.

SELF-TESTS AND EXERCISES FOR PRIME SHOULDERS

Essentially, each one of us has a degree of shoulder mobility that is somewhere on a continuum between hypermobility and close to inflexibility. At the hypermobile end of the scale, the shoulders have no stability. At the other extreme, shoulder muscles are short and inflexible, and joints are stiff.

Have you ever been told that the tops of your shoulders are too tight? Recently, at a lecture I was giving to a number of CEOs and their spouses, I asked that very question. The universal response was "Yes!" They looked at me as if I were psychic. Far from it. In my line of work, patients often tell me that's their problem. What they don't realize is that the problem is not tight muscles but overstretched ones.

Overstretched upper trapezius muscles are much more likely to be a problem than tight ones. If you have shoulders that slope downward and you try to do a lot of stretching for that area, it only makes the problem worse.

Here are some simple self-tests and recommendations to help you adjust your shoulders and keep them in optimum condition.

Lifting Your Arms

Let's begin with a short demonstration that you can do for yourself. Try to reach directly up over your head, lifting your arms as high as you can. Keep your shoulders and shoulder blades down. I predict that you won't be able to get your arms up very high. Many people, especially those of us over 50, will feel some discomfort and limited range of motion.

Now try it a different way. The second time, again reach as high as you can above your head. This time, when you raise your arms, allow your shoulders to rise up as much as feels natural. But don't bring your shoulders all the way up to your ears.

Does the first movement, or the second, feel better? You will probably feel more comfortable when you allow your shoulders to rise. This opens your acromial space—the space between your shoulder blade and your humerus—creating room for the tissues between them and the head of the humerus to rotate up freely.

The objective is to lift your arms without pain and without bringing your shoulders all the way up to your ears.

Do You Have Sloping Shoulders?

Look at yourself in the mirror. Do your collarbones slope down from the inside to the outside of your shoulder? Do you feel tension in your shoulders and neck?

If you have sloping shoulders, avoid stretching the tops of your shoulders. That kind of stretching—which many people try for tension release—actually decreases the subacromial space. For instance, if you stretch the upper trapezius by dropping your head to one side and pressing your opposite shoulder down, you will probably make your shoulders worse. The muscle may, indeed, be "tight," not because it is too short or stiff, but because, in a constant stretch, it is pulled out taut.

For example, if you sling a heavy bag strap over a shoulder, it is stretched down and is extremely "tight." Stretching it more would not help, but hurt.

At all times, try to maintain good shoulder posture—that is, with the shoulders almost level. Lowering your shoulders creates tension in your muscles. Stretching them downward makes the problem worse. People with heavy arms, broad shoulders, and large chest and back muscles are especially prone to this problem.

Remember, if you feel this kind of shoulder pain, it's not coming from *tense* shoulders, but from pinching in the subacromial space (against the tissues within) or from straining an overstretched muscle.

So remind yourself to elevate your shoulders naturally. Do this by maintaining good posture with no tension in your shoulders. When sitting at your desk, use armrests that are high enough to keep your shoulders level. With your elbows supported on high armrests, your upper shoulders are tension free.

Also, don't carry a heavy bag, briefcase, or suitcase suspended from one shoulder by a single strap. If you have an existing shoulder problem, this kind of bag toting will only make the problem worse. I'm very much in favor of suitcases and backpacks that have wheels. Or, better yet, travel light.

Are You Rounding Your Back?

To take care of your shoulders, avoid slumping over or rounding your upper back. A flexed, rounded upper and middle back—which many people acquire with age—is a potential cause of shoulder problems. (There's a good chance the rounded-back problem is caused by short, stiff latissimus dorsi muscles.)

If you can't fully extend your upper back, shoulder movement will suffer. For instance, it's very difficult to raise your arms over your head if your upper back is rounded over. (Just try it and see!)

If you have an impingement, rotator cuff problem, bursitis, or any other shoulder problem, rounding your back is likely to make a familiar pain feel even worse. When you're standing or walking, try to keep a straight upper back, not by straining, but gently, in a relaxed way. When you do, it will be a lot easier to lift your arms over your head, even extending them into a straight, 170- to 180-degree position.

Stretches That Can Help Your Back

If your latissimus dorsi muscles—your "lats"—are short and stiff, they can cause a rounded upper back and contribute in other ways to shoulder problems. (In fact, short, stiff lats relate to a wide range of pain in different parts of the body—including your mid-back, shoulder, neck, and jaw.) They also prevent adequate external rotation of the humerus, which creates impingement.

To help prevent this, perform the "L" stretch (see page 47), the quadruped rock back stretch (see page 48), and the latissimus dorsi stretch.

The simple, powerful quadruped rock back exercise helps you focus on keeping your spine straight and will enable you to have better shoulder mechanics. As you push back with your arms straight, you are engaging your serratus anterior muscles, which function to rotate your shoulder blades in an upward direction. Performed correctly, this exercise should never cause any shoulder discomfort. It stretches short latissimus dorsi, rhomboids, and all of the muscles that resist normal shoulder motion. It also feels good!

MODIFICATION IN WEIGHT TRAINING OR RESISTANCE TRAINING

If you have shoulder problems and you also do weight-training exercises, I recommend that you don't do wide lat pulldowns with an overhand grip. Though this exercise helps produce larger, wider lats, creating the popular V-shaped upper body, it can actually cause impingement. Instead, use an *underhand* grip (as in a chinup), pulling the bar to your chest. This creates more space between the bones, and it promotes better posture. (It works your muscles just as well, and it keeps you supple.)

The underhand grip can be used to stretch the muscles and the space between the joints with every repetition. Always allow the bar to gently pull your arms *up*, stretching the shoulders up. Be sure to use a shoulder-width grip.

With resistance-training exercises such as the lateral shoulder raise and overhead presses, lift up and out in the plane of your scapula. Never reach straight out to your sides. For the correct form, see the lateral shoulder raise exercise (see page 72).

CHAPTER ELEVEN

PAIN . . . LETTING IT GO

"Think about the painful episodes of your life. You know you've left them behind and that you've healed when you can laugh about them."

—*Bob Newhart*

In previous chapters I've described the pain that can be pegged to a particular part of the body. If that body part is injured, abused, or neglected, there are adjustments, exercises, or treatments, as I've shown, that can help alleviate pain. But what if you take these measures and they don't work? What if your pain decreases but won't go away? And what about living with low-level pain, the kind that doesn't respond to exercise or treatment?

For some, the answer is medication. Certainly, some medications are helpful for chronic conditions that make normal activities impossible. But in my experience, I've found that many kinds of pain can be handled without any medication at all. It's a matter of retraining our brains and learning new skills.

Some pain-relief strategies take education. Some others require consistency.

Still others require awareness. For most musculoskeletal conditions, education, consistency, and awareness are *all* necessary for a pain-relief program to work successfully.

OUR INTERNAL PAINKILLERS

Every one of us has a powerful painkilling system within us. Certain opiates reside inside our bodies—compounds with names like enkephalins, dynorphins, and endorphins—that are believed to be more powerful for pain relief than many pharmaceutical painkillers. Medications that relieve pain do so by releasing chemicals that attach to certain "receptor sites" in our neurological system, a process that immediately helps dull the sensation of pain. Our self-made painkillers, the ones produced by our own bodies, work in essentially the same way, honing in on receptor sites when pain fighting begins.

If you've ever helped a sick or an injured child feel better with a gentle touch, comforting words, or a special treat, you realize that the child's internally produced painkillers are your allies. The placebo effect—another way to describe this kind of healing—is not just "in your head." You are capable of turning on the very real pain-relief systems in that child's body. And with practice, you may very well be able to do the same with your own body.

Relieving Your Pain, Boosting Your Mood

One of the proven paths to that kind of pain relief is exercise. Exercise activates our enkephalins and endorphins, two of those internally produced chemicals that are key to pain relief. Even at modest levels of exercise, the pain level tends to decrease and mood improves. It's a phenomenon I've witnessed and experienced many times myself.

Earlier in this book, I referred to the survey that I give participants both before and immediately after classes in the Life Enhancement Center at Canyon Ranch. Among other things, I ask people to give me ratings of their pain levels before and after a workout. (We use a common method—a rating system that ranges from 0 to 10 on a pain scale.) In these classes, the results support what other research has shown. Pain consistently drops, frequently after just one workout.

This is achieved without extraordinary effort and without any exercises targeted to specific problem areas. I encourage the participants to stay at a level of moderate intensity throughout.

If you have any doubts, there's an easy way to find out whether you can confirm these results. Give exercise a chance! The next time you're feeling some pain (or right now, if it's convenient), evaluate your pain on a scale from 0 to 10, with 0 being completely pain free and 10 being the most serious level of pain you have ever experienced. Then go for a brisk walk. When you get back, evaluate your pain level again. See whether you don't feel better afterward.

(Of course, when choosing an exercise, you don't want to aggravate the area that's causing the pain. But as long as you've been cleared to exercise by your therapist or doctor, just choose an exercise that doesn't directly involve the painful area. If you have shoulder pain, walking will help you feel better. If you have knee pain, then swimming or riding a bike—with good alignment—is the better choice.)

Listening to Your Body

Generally, just staying in good shape, using the functional fitness program that I've described in this book, is the best way to keep your "natural painkillers" ready to do their job. When you're *out* of shape, on the other hand, your whole system suffers, and that includes your body's ability to generate internal painkillers. For people who remain sedentary, pain is likely to feel more intense and to last longer.

As you can tell from my previous comments, I'm not one of those gung-ho guys who encourages people to "play through pain." On the contrary, as I have emphasized in every description of prime-for-life strategies, I want you to regard pain as a very important signal. It's your body's alarm system, telling you that something is wrong or about to go wrong. If you're just starting to exercise, learning a sport, or doing a new workout, stay aware. When your body talks to you, listen!

WHAT'S THE REAL STORY OF PAIN?

Pain is a protective mechanism; it is our body's response to tissue damage. Pain elicits a withdrawal response—it makes us want to escape the source of our injury. It is a teacher, educating us about things that harm our bodies. And it is a hard taskmaster.

There are four primary sources of pain:

○ Cutaneous: This refers to pain that involves the skin.

○ Deep somatic: Deep somatic pain arises from injury or something that's gone wrong in our bones, nerves, muscles, tendons, ligaments, or vascular system.

○ Visceral: This is pain that comes from internal organs, such as the lungs, heart, reproductive tissues, etc.

○ Referred: This is when pain originates in a place that is different from where you feel the pain. This happens because the area that hurts may share a nerve with one that innervates some other part of the body. For example, during fetal development, the heart and the left shoulder share the same nerve. Consequently, pain from a heart attack may be felt in the left shoulder or down the arm. Back pain may be a manifestation of disease of the abdomen or pelvis. Or, as I've mentioned, pain caused by the gallbladder may be referred to the right shoulder blade.

Referred pain is common. If you have unrelenting pain that interferes with your daily activities, please see your doctor as soon as possible. You may also opt to see a physical therapist—we deal with many types of pain.

WHERE TO BEGIN FINDING RELIEF

As I've noted, a physical therapist will make a diagnosis based on the mechanical cause of your pain, but we're also trained to screen for issues outside our practice. If your shoulder does not meet the criteria of a movement impairment of the shoulder joint, we refer you to the appropriate clinician.

Somatic pain—pain that is in the joints, muscles, bone, nerves, ligaments, or vascular system—is the most common pain treated by physical therapists. Referred pain from an irritated upper trapezius muscle can cause headaches and disc problems in the spine, or cause radiating pain in the arms or legs; we deal with that, too.

One source of somatic pain is trigger points. These are the small regions of "misbehaving" muscles that I referred to earlier in this book. They are tender to the touch, or sometimes without touch, and refer pain to other places that are predictable. A lot has been written about these localized regions of very irritable and tender points. (President John F. Kennedy's physician, Dr. Janet Travell, was one of the first to thoroughly map out reproducible pain-referral patterns.) Unquestionably, they are a common source for musculoskeletal pain. They often occur at sites where nerves enter the muscles that they control.

Pain Treatments You May Encounter

In your search for a pain-free life, you'll come across many methods that offer relief. Some treatments have been used for years, such as acupuncture or "nee-dling" (putting in a dry needle), electrical stimulation, injection of anesthetic agents, "spray and stretch" (spraying a vaso-coolant on the skin over the region of pain), and applying pressure to the trigger point. It is not clearly understood how each works, but many of these produce good results in some people. For example:

○ Many trigger point locations also correspond to acupuncture points. So patients may get quick relief with an acupuncture treatment.

○ Injection of an anesthetic agent by a physician can also quiet down the region of hyperactivity. (Trigger points may indicate a region of hyperexcitability in that part of a muscle.)

○ "Spray and stretch" involves spraying a cold substance along the course of the muscle, while it is gently stretched. It works.

○ Currently, there are many practitioners in the PT and massage professions who are trained to apply pressure directly to the trigger point. It is believed, but not proven, that squeezing out bloodflow, depriving the area of oxygen, causes a rebound effect of increased bloodflow, but this is only one of many theories about this generally effective technique.

○ Another method used by some PTs is positional release, in which the muscle is passively put into a position of no tension; the two ends of the muscle are brought so close together that all tension is removed for about 90 seconds.

Early in my practice I had remarkable results using positional release and, sometimes, spray and stretch. Patients who arrived in agony would get off the table completely relieved of pain! I used these techniques to eliminate headaches, neck pain, low back pain, and pelvic pain with great success. But I soon realized, as my patients kept returning, that the techniques did not always provide a permanent cure. These techniques, even if only temporary, can provide a significant release from pain.

Getting to the Source

Until recently, all musculoskeletal problems were thought to be caused by restricted tissues—"tight muscles" or "stuck joints"—and releasing tightness seemed to be the cure for every known ailment. Joint manipulation, trigger point release, and/or stretching of the muscles were performed to a fare-thee-well. Sometimes these approaches work.

The cutting edge today? We are recognizing that musculoskeletal pain can be caused by muscles that are too short, too weak, *or* too long. Shirley Sahrmann, PT, PhD, along with one of the giants of the physical therapy world, Florence Kendall, PT, have studied certain muscles, such as the piriformis in the buttocks, and also the area of the upper trapezius, that cause pain when overstretched. Their research shows that the body is far more complicated than we know. It makes evaluating a patient more complex, but when we take the role of muscles into account, it makes for better outcomes.

Pain is subjective, and perception is everything. Pain is affected by stress, fear, fatigue, and deconditioning. Developing strategies for diminishing pain is a necessity, not a luxury.

Strategies for Dealing with Pain Today

We'd like to believe that for every ailment, there's either an immediate cure or one that's waiting just around the corner. If we could only find that Magic Pill or Mystic Healer, life would be smooth sailing! As a physical therapist, however, I have come to believe that pain is part of life. Most of us won't have pain very often, but all of us will undergo pain sometime—emotional or physical. It is as present as joy, birth, and death. I also believe that coping mechanisms are a must for every one of us.

A few years ago I attended an educational seminar on musculoskeletal pain. There were about 40 attendees, half of them physicians and the other half physical therapists. If anyone knew about treating pain, it was this group. But when the presenter asked by a show of hands how many of us were experiencing some level of pain at that time, at least half of the participants raised their hands. Including me. I was experiencing some pain from an injury sustained in a minor bicycling accident.

There's a lesson for us here. Pain is a bad experience, but we survive it. Pain is a physical sensation, but *we* are not *the pain*—it's something *separate* from us.

Now, at the age of 59, I've learned to deal with periodic pain. Have I had more than other people? Not by a long shot. I've worked with people who have experienced far worse pain than I have ever known. As a physical therapist, I've worked with terminal patients in geriatric hospitals and nursing homes. I've performed wound care on individuals with enormous, gaping wounds. I'm one of the lucky ones because I have been able to develop skills and use resources to deal with pain when I've had it. Others are not so fortunate, and for some it may be impossible. But all of us are well served by learning more about the origins of pain and developing our own ways to deal with it.

Pain Medication for Your Joints and Bones

Many common medications for musculoskeletal pain are falling out of favor with the physicians here at Canyon Ranch. These medications are nonsteroidal anti-inflammatory drugs, NSAIDS, and they are part of a "family" that includes aspirin, ibuprofen, and naproxen. They've been used for decades to treat ankle pain, headaches, muscle soreness, muscle and joint injuries—just about everything imaginable.

Because many NSAIDs are nonprescription drugs, you can pick them up in a drugstore and take them without any medical advice. Directions are on the label. They are wonderful drugs for many reasons. Using them, however, has its risks. NSAIDs have been implicated in a *New England Journal of Medicine* article in more than 16,000 deaths annually in the United States, primarily in cases where they were implicated in gastrointestinal bleeding.

Cox-2 inhibitors such as Celebrex and Vioxx were developed to provide pain relief without irritating the gastrointestinal lining. They were meant to avoid the risk of gastrointestinal bleeding that NSAIDs carry. Then studies showed these newer drugs carried the potential of increasing risk of heart failure in some individuals.

What's the Best Policy?

Obviously, I advise taking a measured approach when it comes to pain relief. This is not a call for a return to the days when people were told to "buck up and take it." Many of us experience pain that is debilitating and saps the joy out of our lives. But history has also shown that today's miracle drug may be tomorrow's nightmare, so we must be cautious when we use medications for pain relief.

OVER-THE-COUNTER DRUGS AND YOU

Even though over-the-counter drugs (OTCs) do not require a prescription, they do carry potential risks. One of the most popular, when it comes to relieving pain, is acetaminophen (with brand names such as Tylenol). It does not decrease inflammation, but it does help with pain relief. However, it is also linked to liver failure. (In one study of emergency room reports from four different hospitals in Virginia, for instance, acetaminophen was indicated as a leading cause of acute liver failure.)

Common NSAIDS such as aspirin and ibuprofen are also available without prescription. As I've noted, they have been associated with gastrointestinal bleeding, and can have other harmful effects as well. For example, NSAIDs have been implicated in poor healing of bones, tendons, and muscles.

A 1995 study looked at the effect of NSAIDs on muscle regeneration in rats after these animals had exercise-induced muscle damage (the damage was roughly the equivalent of what you get when you're sore several days after a downhill hike). The group of rats that were given NSAIDs did not have a complete regeneration of healthy muscle tissue. If the same holds for humans, then taking aspirin or ibuprofen for muscle soreness may be counterproductive. Pain is decreased, but so is healing. Researchers have suggested that muscle actually *requires* an inflammatory phase before it can get stronger and heal.

This is not to say you should *never* take any pain medications. Your doctor is an expert in management of medication issues. But Americans tend to reflexively use over-the-counter medications, thinking they are always harmless. Clearly, this is not so.

When it comes to the discomfort caused by exercise, I think it's important to be aware of what you should expect. I've previously described delayed onset muscle soreness (DOMS) that is just a normal part of exercise. Ease in gently, but if you do get DOMS, wait it out—it will pass. You really don't need to use a pain-relieving medication for DOMS.

Another way to avoid pain—as I've mentioned repeatedly—is to prevent it in the first place. Hard work is sometimes part of exercise. But you're better off stopping when you feel pain, especially joint pain, rather than counting on an over-the-counter drug afterward to help "fix" the pain. (It won't!)

I also advise people to try finding alternative paths to pain relief. And keep searching. Why take medication, for instance, if you haven't tried rest, ice, compression, and elevation (the RICE technique described on page 114)? As I've seen myself on numerous occasions, there really are many alternatives that can be tried before asking your physician for pain medications.

But . . . having said all that, if you have horrendous pain, sometimes you do what you must. See your doctor. Be thankful for the miraculous drugs out there!

WHAT CAN LAUGHTER DO FOR YOU?

You've heard it before: Laughter is a natural analgesic. Not only that, but it can also be *powerful* medicine.

In one study, researchers measured the effect of laughter on the pain threshold of a number of subjects. There were two groups in the study, and everyone in both groups was assigned to hold their hands submerged as long as possible in painfully cold water. One group had no distractions. The other group watched funny movies and, naturally, laughed at lot at the funny parts.

Turns out, the laughing participants tolerated the discomfort of cold water significantly longer.

Some years later, researchers repeated the study. This time, they did blood tests to find out whether there were any hormonal changes (detectable in the blood) when the two groups were tested in the same way. They found that the laughing subjects not only withstood the cold water longer, but they also handled the stress differently.

The "laughter" group had significantly less of the stress hormone cortisol than the "serious" group. Apparently, they did not register the pain as being stressful while they were laughing. (The group in the quiet, somber room had quite a different experience.)

Will laughter alone make pain go away? Obviously not. But as this study shows, your perception of pain has a real effect on body chemistry.

Here's an example of that. Suppose you go to your doctor with complaints of shoulder pain. After a series of x-rays and tests, he tells you that you have a bruised muscle, suggests that you ice it, and tells you it will probably be gone in a few days. Obviously, there's little to fear in a scenario like this, and it's likely that you'll perceive this as a fairly minor pain. But now imagine another scenario—that you go to the doctor with the same complaint and are told that your pain is symptomatic of a life-threatening tumor. The mild, nagging discomfort has turned into a reminder of your mortality. Fear, immediately, magnifies your pain.

Again, this response is not just "in your head." There are physiological effects. Fear activates the primitive fight-or-flight response—that heart-pounding, adrenalin-pumping response that we have when we're in terrible danger. Your cortisol levels shoot up. Fear increases muscle tension, increases blood pressure, and gets your mind racing at a thousand miles per hour as you frantically think of an escape route. It is the opposite response of calm.

The bottom line: Pain is mediated by your perception of it.

So, when dealing with pain, it is *essential* to find the ways that work best for you to dispel fear, seek calm, and bolster your immune system at the same time.

Randy's
STORY

Yes, this is about me. And the story really starts when I first began to read the work of news magazine editor and author Norman Cousins. In his book *Anatomy of an Illness*, published in 1979, Cousins wrote about saving his own life with laughter. He had a potentially terminal illness and, regardless of what his horde of doctors tried, he kept getting worse. Checking himself into a hotel, Cousins created his own recipe for healing—a complete set of Marx Brothers movies. With this as his "medicine," Cousins said, he actually laughed his way back to good health.

In my case, I didn't have the Marx Brothers. But I did have the movie *Airplane*. Thinking back on my own experience, I'm quite sure that movie helped save my life in much the same way as the Marx Brothers rescued Norman Cousins.

I'd been working at a resort in Mexico and was felled by dysentery. I mean felled. For 5 lost days, I was unconscious and delirious in a San Diego hospital. When discharged, I still couldn't eat.

The resident who discharged me said the virulent organism ravaging my gut would take between 7 and 10 days to pass through. He gave me three cases of Gatorade for electrolyte replacement and encouraged me to eat a banana or bowl of cooked rice every day.

"Sometimes this becomes chronic, but it rarely kills," the resident said in parting. "Don't worry. You'll be fine if you can hold down solid food during the next 10 days."

My family was back east, and I was young. I had no idea that life was so tenuous. For 5 days in that San Diego hospital, I'd been on an intravenous diet. Now I was returning to Mexico, where I was consigned to a rickety shanty, away from guests and other staff. I had a hot plate that I used to cook my own rice. Every day, as soon as I ate it, the rumbling started and I'd stumble weakly to the john. I couldn't even keep the Gatorade down.

Day 15 arrived. I still couldn't eat. Occasionally a sympathetic employee would pop in and tell me to "think positive." (Later, staff members told me they thought that encouragement was my only hope for survival.)

I was depressed, alone, very ill, in another country. And I was unable to get well. Finally, in desperation, I dressed and made the journey out to my car. Although the car was parked only a quarter mile from my hut, that trek seemed to take forever. I had to make numerous rest stops. I think I cried when I finally reached the car and climbed in. To my infinite relief, the engine turned over immediately.

I drove across the border and went to a movie. *Airplane* was on the marquee. I assumed it was some kind of war movie or adventure film. I didn't care—I just wanted to take my mind off my illness and sit in the dark.

Soon the nonstop, corny jokes had me howling with laughter. The humor was a counterpoint to my misery, and with the laughter came an incredible flood of relief. When I walked outside, I was still laughing out loud. There was a thermos of rice in my car. I ate it and I knew that I was going to be okay. That rice was the best meal I've ever had. And I got better.

I believe the joy sparked by that slapstick movie saved my life.

Norman Cousins, I believe you! Laughter heals.

ACTIVATE YOUR INTERNAL HEALING SYSTEM

Relaxing activities can kick-start your parasympathetic system and decrease pain. These activities include favorite hobbies, especially music and art, working in the garden (or even sitting there, breathing it all in), and any form of play.

And hang out with kids whenever you can. A lot of times kids are fun and uncomplicated to be around. They remind us of the simple causes of joy and laughter.

When we bought our house, I replicated one of the most relaxing and nurturing rituals of my childhood. Every summer I used to visit my Aunt Teddy, deep in the Blue Ridge Mountains of Virginia. Teddy was the closest thing to a grandparent I had. I loved her. She had a wooden porch swing hanging from the high beams on her porch. Sitting with her at twilight—talking, drinking, watching fireflies come out, and waving at the Walters family (on the other side of the street) through the weeping willows—those memories are nurturing, treasured, and magical. The gentle rocking, creaking, and talking relaxed me to the inside of my bones.

I have a porch swing now, and the magic still works. It's nice to rock, look at

TURNING OFF YOUR MIND

Do you want to try to experience meditation? You don't have to check into a quiet temple or take lessons from a master. Although it helps to have "guided meditation"—led by someone who can take you through the steps of being in the moment—you can also try it by yourself, in the privacy of your own home. Here's what you do:

● Choose a quiet room (your bedroom is fine) where you won't be disturbed for a while. Set the alarm for 20 minutes. Lie on your back with a rolled blanket under your knees and a low, soft pillow under your head. Let your body be comfortable, with your arms and legs in a relaxed position, symmetrically placed on either side of your body. Close your eyes.

● Starting with your toes, focus on relaxing each part of your body. Let your concentration move gradually from your toes to your head. When you reach your head, be specific about each part of the head you're focusing on. Linger on your scalp, forehead, eyes, jaws, lips, tongue, and throat. Finally, go inside to your breath. Pay attention to your inhalations. Let each breath become as shallow as it wishes to be. Imagine the air doing the work for you.

● Let your thoughts drift—don't try to stop them. Each time a thought arises, let it float to the surface, as if you were in still water and the thought were a bubble. Then let it go.

● Next, give attention to the still, brief moments in your breathing between exhaling and inhaling. In that still moment, you will find a nanosecond of no-thought. Don't struggle to hold it—simply acknowledge it. Don't try to stop the thoughts that keep floating like bubbles to the surface of your mind. Simply let them go. Let go of the tension in your body. Exhale everything out into the world around you.

● There is nothing to do now, nothing to accomplish. Quietly give your attention to the stillness of the moments between thoughts.

our garden, admire the beauty of our home, and, once in a while, remember my Aunt Teddy. We need to start saying "No" to the constant stimulation of television, radio, MP3 players, and ringing cell phones. We need to say "Yes" to creaking porch swings and stars. Appreciation is surely one element of natural healing.

Touch—The Hormone of Love

Our skin is meant to touch and to be touched. Whether it's the hug of a friend, holding a child's hand, or the miracle of sexuality, touch calms us and allows us to feel nurtured. We have a neurotransmitter called oxytocin that lowers blood pressure and increases feelings of well-being. Oxytocin is called the hormone of love because it increases with touch, massage, and orgasms. Its concentration in the body was found to correlate to lower blood pressure. And it rises—research has shown—when we express feelings of love toward others. Sometimes oxytocin is given to new mothers to help their breast milk flow.

So—add touch to your life. We are animals well designed to lead prime and happy lives if we're willing. Hug those you love, hold a hand, or caress your loved one.

Prayer—A Metaphor for Love

Prayer is a universal aid that can help relieve every kind of pain imaginable. Whether you believe in God or not, it's comforting to feel part of something larger than yourself—part of the cosmos. Pain is isolating; prayer is the opposite. It is connection.

Some people who believe in God scoff at nonbelievers, saying, "Right. When the chips are down, they start praying." So what? Even for nonbelievers, God can be a metaphor for love. What harm can there be in reaching out to the infinite in search of comfort? And perhaps there is a great deal of good.

Each Moment Meditation

Meditation is a powerful way to deactivate our fight-or-flight response. Every culture or religion has some form of meditation. A Catholic priest I used to know said, "Meditation is the listening side of prayer rather than the asking side of prayer." I still think it is beautiful, and it is true.

I believe the manifestation of our fight-or-flight response, the ultimate human defense, may be our racing minds. While our wondrous minds can create inventions, discover cures, and find solutions, the same brain cells can also prevent us from experiencing the miracle of each moment.

So how do we keep our minds from racing?

Try going for a walk and keeping your mind on each moment. See each turn of the path, every leaf falling from a tree, the color of water running down the gutters. Listen to that water gurgling and singing. At first, when you try this, you'll likely find you are rarely there. Instead, you're mulling over a meeting you have, balancing your mental checkbook, or rehashing an argument with your spouse. Most beginning meditators say they just can't stay in the moment. But with practice, you can "return to the moment" and stay there. For many, that's a new experience.

When I teach meditation for stress management at Canyon Ranch, there is at least one person after class who says, "I can't stop thinking." I tell them that between each thought is a pause—a nanosecond of stillness. All it takes is acknowledging those fleeting moments of silence. It just takes practice. After a while, you'll look forward to the times you are free from thoughts. They are mini vacations. They begin as fleeting moments and grow.

Pain without Suffering

The little moments of stillness are about being alive in the miracle of the moment. As alive as you will ever be.

Years ago, a Buddhist friend said to me, "Meditation takes a split second to work. The discipline is waiting for the split second to happen."

There's a favorite meditation I do with guests who come to the Life Enhancement Program. When they're lying comfortably on their backs, ready to begin meditation, I ask, "With a show of hands, how many of you have had more pain at other times in your life than you're having right now?"

Every hand goes up.

"How many of you can tolerate the discomforts you might experience in this position for the next 20 minutes?"

They laugh and raise their hands.

Then I say, "Good. Let's try something. For the next 20 minutes, I'd like you *not to move a muscle*. Don't fidget. You've already told me you could tolerate any discomforts that come up in the next 20 minutes. I'd like you to hold on to that."

Now they know we're up to something.

"Fidgeting," I tell them, "is about trying to be in the next moment rather than accepting the present one. Every sensation—your itchy nose, scratchy throat, uncomfortable low back—is less discomfort than you've had during other times in your life."

I lead them through a guided meditation, lingering on each part of their body so they fully experience it. Rarely does someone fidget. It's okay if they do, but then they let go and come back to the present.

Meditation is about choosing to be here now rather than daydreaming. You learn you can tolerate certain levels of discomfort. You also learn there is a difference between pain and suffering. This is more than a mere philosophical concept. When you learn to separate fear from pain, you can experience significant pain without suffering. You come to realize that pain is merely a sensation like others.

MAKING A CHOICE

I believe you can *choose* whether pain will have power over you. In fact, I've had experiences in my own life that (unfortunately) forced me to put that theory to the test.

Several years ago I was at a resort with my beautiful wife and our teenaged son. I went out windsurfing and took a bad fall. The mast crashed down, lacerating my forehead.

Back on shore, I knew I needed stitches. The doctor apologized because he didn't have Novocain—he'd have to stitch me up without the benefit of an anesthetic. This occurred at a time when I'd been practicing meditation for a number of years, and I realized that this procedure would be a good test of my ability to practice what I'd learned. Could I regard pain like that—the pain of a needle stitching very sensitive flesh—as only a sensation, something to be experienced? As a boy, I'd been terrified of any kind of pain. I couldn't even handle shots without writhing and screaming. Would my reaction be that much different now?

Of course, it's difficult to describe exactly what happened when the doctor began to suture the wound. All I can say is that meditation did make a difference—a great difference, in fact. It hurt when the doctor sewed me up. But the pain was only a sensation. I experienced the sensation, but not the terror and not the suffering.

My experience is far from unique.

Research studies have consistently shown that mindfulness meditation—in which one simply focuses on sensations in the body as I've described here—helps people with chronic pain of all kinds. One study of 90 chronic pain patients found that 10 weeks of this activity significantly decreased pain, regardless of the type of pain the person had.

Another study of 37 chronic low back pain sufferers aged 65 or older produced similar results. More than eight out of 10 participants who meditated for about half an hour, for 4 or 5 days out of every week, found that their acceptance of pain dramatically improved. And along with that, they were more mobile and functioned better in their daily lives. They had learned to separate pain from suffering.

Attitude and Pain

In the early '90s, I took a leave from Canyon Ranch and commuted 500 miles each week to attend physical therapy classes at Northern Arizona University. My wife and son were in Tucson. At the end of that grueling time, I got a job working in a hospital with people who were seriously ill.

I remember two women quite well. One had been in a car accident and had to have her feet amputated. She would be fitted with prosthetics, but in order to take the pressure, she needed to have therapy to toughen up the ends of her limbs. I, or a physical therapy assistant, would wheel her between the parallel bars and ask her to stand for as long as she could tolerate the pain.

My other patient was a woman who'd suffered a devastating stroke. One side of her body was flaccid and unresponsive, and her face drooped. When she could speak, her words were slurred and halting.

Both women had a long road ahead, and both used the parallel bars at the same time, facing each other. The bars were long enough for them to see each other, but they couldn't hear each other. The woman who'd lost her feet was checking out the woman who had a stroke. She looked at me and whispered, "Seeing her, I realize how lucky I am. She has it so much worse than I do . . . I feel thankful." That was something I hadn't expected to hear.

The next day, my assistant and I switched patients. As I worked with the woman who'd suffered a stroke, I saw her watching the other woman—she was obviously in a lot of pain. My patient mumbled something several times. Then I got it. She said, "Lucky. Luckier than her."

Each woman expressed her gratitude for having been given her own trial—each woman considered herself luckier than the other person. Now that they were ready to tackle their own particular challenges, therapy began to progress faster for both of them. Both expressed to me that they were in deep pain—physical, emotional, and spiritual. Their moment of insight, realizing that they could handle their pain, was a turning point in their respective progress in therapy. They both started smiling again.

None of us gets out of this life without pain. That's a given. I hope that if you are in pain now or ever, you remember that life can still have meaning and joy.

CHAPTER TWELVE

MAKING A PLAN YOU WANT TO LIVE WITH . . . EVERY SINGLE DAY

"You are one workout away
from feeling better."

—*Randy Raugh*

More than a few guests at Canyon Ranch have heard me tell the story of my first aerobic experience. It occurred when I was 5 years old, back in the days when I introduced myself as "Wandy Wow" (I couldn't say my Rs!). One early autumn evening my next-door neighbor Derrick and his sister Belinda came over. They asked my sister and me if we could come outside and play Hookey the Goblin. My parents agreed, and my sister and I flew out the door. I had no idea what "Hookey" meant, but I wanted to find out.

A harvest-orange moon lit the sky. The cool air held the faint scent of smoke from the pile of leaves my dad had been burning. Although I didn't know the rules of Hookey the Goblin, it didn't take long to find out. Soon all of us were chasing each other round and round the yard, screaming, laughing, and scaring each other until we could run no more.

There it is—my first aerobic workout, and it's still a wonderful memory.

When I tell this story, it's not for the sake of boring my guests (though it may do that) or providing a revealing autobiography. I have a point to make, the same one I made at the start of this book. I'd love for all of us to be able to restore the memories as well as the *experience* of movement, with all the thrills of joy and abandonment we felt as kids.

Often the telling of this story strikes a responsive chord in my listeners. The guests at the Ranch, many of whom may have just signed up for their first Life Enhancement class, soon recall the things they liked to do as kids. Before long, I'm hearing about their favorite sports and games, about an outdoor-adventure experience that was unforgettable, or an exhausting and thrilling youthful adventure. They tell me about childhood games that went on so long they seemed never to end. About neighborhood kids who would rush to the diamond, the basketball court, or the soccer field on a summer evening and play until the sun went down.

Too often, of course, these recollections come back in the form of wistful memories of things that happened way too long ago. For some people, there are no comparable experiences filling in the gap of years between right now and back then. But their stay at the Ranch helps remind them of what it feels like to thrive with the joy of movement. And when they've rediscovered how enjoyable an outdoor walk can be or they've come out of a workout class completely "pumped" and ready for more, I try to help them figure out how they can integrate functional fitness into their lives moving forward.

We work it out together. We come up with a plan. It's a plan that takes into account the limitations on their time, their obligations of work and family, the unexpected changes in schedule, the many contingencies that can interfere with them getting the exercise they want and need. It's also a plan that acknowledges how each body works, how much attention it needs, and its requirements for high-energy workouts and rest and relaxation.

In developing a functional fitness plan for each individual, we talk about the emotional reasons for exercise. We recall, from what we have done during the previous week, how good it feels to exercise and how great we feel afterward. We reignite the flame of enthusiasm that we had when we were kids—the eagerness to dash around after goblins, hide behind trees, run for a loose ball, or roll down a grassy lawn.

So, now that you know what's involved, let's work out a plan for you.

STEP ONE: DON'T PRESSURE YOURSELF (KICK GUILT OUT THE DOOR!)

If you engage in a more active life, you will reap all the benefits spelled out in this book, including more joy. If you want to move more but don't know how to start, here's the first step: Don't pressure yourself.

We live in an "-aholic" culture. We are alcoholics, couch-potatoaholics, rageaholics, rushaholics, sexaholics, workaholics, and all of it is killing us. So . . . I don't want exercise to become another obsession that eats you alive! Can you, instead, befriend exercise and dance with it?

I would like you to use exercise as a time to create more inner space, freedom, joy, and radiant health. Take the pressure off. Delight in movement.

As you prime for life, look for the middle ground. This is the path to sustained physical and emotional health. It is the path to making and keeping a plan that works. It also allows you flexibility. Yes, you can change your exercise routine when life changes. I want your life to be better, not more burdensome.

I hereby declare that you can allow yourself to be free of pressure.

STEP TWO: REMEMBER EXPERIENCES OF JOYFUL MOVEMENT

How do you feel about exercise now? Do you think it is dull, boring, and painful, or fun, enlivening, and energizing?

Step two is remembering past experiences of joyful movement. When you lose interest in exercise, recall those moments. You can make a list (some people do well with lists). Or keep a journal. Or store information inside your head. Whichever is your way—that's the right way.

Your list of good memories of movement can be as long or as short as you want. Here are some of my own great memories that get me moving and keep me moving. I want to share them here, hoping they'll spark your imagination or bring up some of your own good memories.

○ I remember the time I passed my deep-water swimming test. I was 6 years old, and I finally got to go into the deep end of the pool. I was scared of jumping off the diving board, but I looked over at my dad, and he gave me a nod of encouragement. When he did that, I had to try.

The kid behind me said, "Hurry up, it's my turn." Excited but terrified, I stepped to the edge and jumped. I felt myself falling into the unknown in slow motion. Then there was the splash—me, landing in the water! I swam to the edge of the pool, and quickly climbed out. I'd made it! Without a moment's hesitation, I headed for the diving board again.

All day long, I dove and swam. I never wanted that day to end. Water was an exciting, new world. When I opened my eyes, I was a frogman!

Every day of my sixth summer I was the first one in, and the last one out of, the pool. I still remember the wonderful smell of chlorine on a warm afternoon and all its associations. And I still love swimming.

○ I remember afternoons at the Tierneys' house. All the neighborhood kids gathered there. The house was warm and the yard outside was great to play in. Big kids and little kids played together—age didn't matter. I was about 9 years old then, somewhere in the middle of the crowd. We'd play hard, running and laughing. Finally, the sun would begin to set, the sky would turn colors, and the fireflies would come out. I'd lie in the grass with my friend Lizzard. Deliciously tired, we'd share our deepest secrets, hopes, and desires. Play would bring us together and clean us out, through and through. In that miraculous time, I felt that life couldn't get any better.

○ I'm in my canoe, gliding 22 miles down the upper Allegheny River, past wading herons and an occasional fisherman. There's the smell of a river, rich and bubbling over gray-blue stones. I was becoming a young man. My friend and I would stop once in a while to jump into the river and cool off, then paddle some more. The river guide would holler, "Rapids ahead!" With heart pounding, eyes wide with anticipation, we frantically paddled, yelling, "Watch out for that rock!" We ran that roiling, turbulent rapid, and it was a moment of being alive, full of joy.

O I used to take backpacking trips in West Virginia. With one companion or another, I hiked the woods, exploring new trails. It's another world. There are animal tracks crossing the path. Silence wraps the trees. One day a deer walked into my camp, came within 6 feet, and kept me company for 10 minutes before it wandered off.

I remember drinking sweet, spring water. Alone and free in an unnamed paradise, I was entranced by each new turn in the trail. I felt good about finding a place that could only be found while walking. I huffed and puffed up dark forest trails across a primitive rope-and-wood footbridge into an area of mystery and solitude. When I lay on a large, warm rock along a river, taking a breather, I daydreamed and was at peace with myself and the world. It was the walking that made it special, and the walking that made me want to do more.

O I took up running at age 22. Initially, it was a way to help me hike all day long without tiring. I knew the stronger and fitter my body was, the more I'd experience. I wanted to be confident that I could make it up a hill without feeling miserable. So I started running to get strong. Running made hiking even more pleasurable, and then I began enjoying the act of running for its own sake.

O As I entered my fifties, I started to choose other types of exercise so I wouldn't hurt my knees. (Much as I enjoy it, running takes a toll on the knees, and I want to be active the rest of my life.) I enjoy stationary bikes, Nordic Track machines, rowing machines, elliptical trainers—you name it.

O And, always, there are walks. Always.

I believe in new beginnings. My wife Lynne and I both work at Canyon Ranch. Not long ago, for our 25th working anniversary, Canyon Ranch gave us new mountain bikes. Do you remember your first bike? What greater pleasure is there than a new bicycle? I have good news for you. The pleasure doesn't change with age. I am as excited about this bike as I was when I got my very first bike. Use your sense of joy to guide your exercise plans.

When is it time for you to start a new form of exercise? That's up to you, of course, but don't be surprised if you're initially bored with the new exercise. That happens to me—and invariably, I discover my boredom is due to a lack of fitness for that activity. So, when you take up a new exercise, stick with it long enough to really give it a chance. You may discover that it makes you feel good and is enjoyable, too.

STEP THREE: FINDING YOUR PERSONAL JOY

If you are not moving enough now, what will it take to help you start living a more active life?

Explore how exercise and movement make you feel—before and after. First of all, copy the next page a few times. Think of some types of exercise, movement, or play that you might like to try. It could be a half-hour walk up the hill behind your house, an exercise class, or a game of tennis. Your self-assignment is to perform 30 minutes of *something* and evaluate your responses before and after.

Before you begin the activity you've chosen, fill out one of the copies of the "Before/After Exercise Feeling Inventory." Circle the number that reflects how you feel about each of the six categories. For example, if you don't want to work out at all, circle the number 1. If you can hardly wait to start, circle the number 5. In other words, 1 reflects *the least* and 5 *the most* for each category.

At the bottom of the form, you are asked to calibrate your current level of pain. If you have no pain, circle the zero. If you are experiencing the most pain you can imagine, circle the number 10.

(Reminder: Whatever activity you choose, make sure it's *not* an exercise that would increase pain in the area where you're feeling it. Select an activity that works something *other* than the painful area and make sure you've been cleared by your MD or PT.)

Immediately after finishing your 30 minutes of activity, fill out the form again. Circle the number that reflects how you feel at that moment. Do it without looking back at your first "Before/After Exercise Feeling Inventory."

Now circle the number from 6 to 20 that reflects, on average, how hard you exercised during the session. (For this, I have provided the Borg Perceived Exertion Scale that I introduced you to earlier, on page 254.) Then write something down that you enjoyed about the activity. This might be a feeling you experienced during the activity such as pride, being glad you finished, pleasure in some movement, a view on the walk, a discovery of your ability . . . the sky is the limit. (Maybe you rediscovered the color of sky!)

What about this exercise session did you enjoy the most (i.e., emotionally, physically, visually, etc.)?

BEFORE/AFTER EXERCISE FEELING INVENTORY

Date:_____

Circle the number that describes how you feel **right now**.

	LEAST				MOST
I feel like working out/ I'm glad I did	1	2	3	4	5
I feel like working out	1	2	3	4	5
Tired	1	2	3	4	5
Calm	1	2	3	4	5
Energetic	1	2	3	4	5
Enthusiastic	1	2	3	4	5
Happy	1	2	3	4	5
Pain	0 1 3 4 5 6 7 8 9 10				

Please do not look at this again after completing it.

BORG PERCEIVED EXERTION SCALE

Circle the number that best represents how hard you were working during exercise.

6	Sitting in a chair..
7	Very, very light intensity ....
8	....
9	Very light intensity..
10	....
11	Fairly light intensity (can converse in long sentences) ....
12	....
13	Somewhat hard intensity (can speak in short sentences)
14	....
15	Hard intensity (can speak only phrases and feel breathless)
16	....
17	Very hard intensity ....
18	....
19	Very, very hard intensity..
20	Maximal exertion ....

After you complete the second "Before/After Exercise Feeling Inventory," compare your responses, question by question, to the first "Before/After Exercise Feeling Inventory." If you indicated that you didn't particularly want to exercise, did you see a change? Did you feel energized afterward? Perhaps you had *less* energy? (If you still feel tired an hour later, you probably exercised too intensely.)

If you had pain at the beginning, did it change? Usually it diminishes. If not, you probably had improper alignment and may want to read the chapter that covers the joint that's bothering you. You could have an injury that needs addressing. You may need to lighten up or choose a better activity for your body.

Through years of using this inventory, I have found that if people go over 16 on the Borg Scale, they may not feel as good after exercise unless they are very fit and used to high intensity. For most of us, staying at "moderate" is conducive to regular exercise. Which is better? A small success or a big failure? Please, give yourself permission to succeed.

Use these inventories for a while as a reminder that exercise does make you feel better. They're also helpful for keeping track of which exercises make you feel particularly good! (But don't make a chore of this. The "inventory" is simply a tool to help you!)

Also remember: Regular exercisers don't usually do it for the long-term benefits. They exercise because they have come to realize this truth:

You are one workout away from feeling better.

CONSIDERATIONS FOR PUTTING YOUR PLAN TOGETHER

There a few things to keep in mind as you develop a program that works for you. Refer back to them as you make progress and adjust accordingly.

Start with a Goal—Gently

People often forget that their personal successes were built on a series of baby steps. Think right now of some achievement you've had in your life—an award won, a job attained, an academic program completed, a child successfully raised. Remember how you started. Probably you started with a very small step, perhaps with trepidation about failing. Every day you did a little more. With growing ability, you also had an increase in your feeling of accomplishment. Every journey begins with a single step.

Begin now with a clear, achievable goal. Choose a goal that you're able to reach and want to reach—not one that you *should* reach. If 30 minutes seems too long right now, start with three 10-minute sessions. (Reminder for beginning exercisers: Studies show that people who engage in three short sessions get the same benefits as those who have one 30-minute session.)

Take 10,000 Steps

Buy yourself a pedometer—a simple, cheap one that only counts steps. (You don't need the kind that translates into miles based upon step length, and besides, these are notoriously inaccurate.) Test your pedometer for a few days to find out how many steps you average in a typical day.

Despite my position as a fitness director, my day-to-day work is often fairly sedentary. I lecture, provide physical therapy consultations, and supervise other people's exercise plans and goals. On a typical day, I take about 6,500 steps. But my goal is 10,000 steps a day! Still, it's not that hard to make up the difference. An evening spent walking our dogs will do it.

Of course, doing the exercises that I love also adds to my total workout. When you know how many steps you take each day, just increase that number by 5 to 10 percent next week, and multiply it by 7.

Example: If you walked 3,000 steps today and average 21,000 steps per week, then next week you can only add between 1,050 and 2,100 more steps, total, for the week. (Increase by no more than 5 to 10 percent of your weekly total, not your daily total.) If it's easier for you, then measure and increase your movement in terms of time instead of number of steps. You are on your way!

Keep Your Exercise Light to Moderate . . . with an Occasional Higher Intensity Session to Spice It Up

The real joys begin when you can work (or play) at a moderate intensity. Make it pleasant. Warm up slowly, and then ease into light intensity for 20 minutes. Slow down for 5 minutes to cool down. Finish with a few minutes of stretches. Remember, at light intensity you should be able to speak in long sentences without sounding slightly out of breath.

After several weeks, put the pedal to the metal and work at a pleasant, moderate rate of intensity. At this intensity, you can only speak in short sentences and might sound slightly breathy, but you could tell your life story. When you enjoy regular exercise sessions, add a few moments of higher intensity—"hard" on the Borg Perceived Exertion Scale—in the middle of your workout two or three times a week.

Add Strength Training

Add strength training slowly. Spend a month in Phase 1. Then ease up to Phase 2. After you can perform 15 repetitions at a given resistance for several workouts, then increase the resistance. Only perform one set of each exercise for a few months. This is enough to improve your muscular fitness.

Spend 3 months in Phase 2. Work hard on increasing repetitions and resistance.

You will love Phase 3. You get to reward yourself for a job well done by not changing anything about it. Your muscles adapt to the new resistance level you attained, and you cruise. This routine can usually be done totally in 10 to 20 minutes. The fitter you become, the faster you go through it.

Phase 4 is designed to increase strength and bone density much more effectively. By the end of it, you'll be doing two sets of each exercise.

Always warm up for 10 minutes first by walking briskly or doing your cardiovascular activity. This prepares your heart and muscles for the work.

While research shows that fairly heavy resistance is needed to build bone density and strength, your ability to lift weight is all relative to your size, age, and genetic ability. The most important element is being patient. Focus on being a little healthier each week. This is about making your life better, and doing it in a way you'll enjoy.

WHAT CAN GET IN YOUR WAY?

When you begin exercising, it's easy to go overboard. At this point in the reading of this book, I know you're probably pumped up about feeling fit—truly alive and prime for the rest of your life. That feeling will stay with you. But like anyone, you will have relapses, times when you stop exercising. When that happens, accept it as part of the program. Do not get down on yourself. Just get moving.

What else gets in the way of exercising? I can name quite a few things, and you can, too. Work, travel, injuries, low energy, food deprivation, sleep deprivation, alcohol, and even caffeine. Many of these factors, separately or combined, can become reasons to stop exercising or to prevent you from starting. So . . . let's see what can be done.

Work

We can't stop working, of course, but here's one thing that people often forget: Sometimes we allow work to become an impediment because we feel righteous about working. I believe everyone has a sanity threshold of work hours. If you step over that threshold, you will short-circuit your exercise plans and everything else. Relaxation, mealtime, and family time—along with work—are all important. So is exercise!

Travel

When you travel to a new time zone, I recommend that you reset your watch as soon as you board the plane. Upon arrival, get on the new time as fast as you can. Get up at your usual time (in the new time zone) and expose yourself to daylight in the morning to reset your circadian rhythms. Eat breakfast at breakfast time in the *new time*, even if it's 3 a.m. at home.

If you're staying in a hotel or motel that doesn't have a gym, exercise by walking. Explore. (Of course, always inquire about safety in the area where you'll be walking.) Most fitness centers and gyms will provide a temporary visitor pass for a reasonable amount of money.

Take your Xertubes in your suitcase and perform your strength exercises. Walk in the airport while waiting for your flight. Use travel as an opportunity to make movement exciting.

Injuries

Active people do get injuries. If this happens, switch to a type of exercise that won't exacerbate your injury. If you're a walker recovering from an ankle sprain, for instance, go swimming instead. Just go easy when you push off the walls of the pool during turns. (You'll usually do fine on a stationary bike, too.)

After injury, when resuming exercise, test gently. If you feel pain, find something else to do. A swimmer's painful shoulder will be irritated by overhead movements such as swimming the crawl, but you can always put on a buoyancy belt and jog in the deep water, or power walk in shallow water. Or you may want to use a rowing machine, beginning slowly, until your shoulder feels better. In other words, there's usually some way to exercise gently when you have a joint injury without aggravating it.

Low Energy

"Lack of energy" is the reason many people give for not exercising. My response is to remind people how exercise *increases* energy rather than diminishing it. If you find that you're more tired after exercising than you were before, it probably means you've done too much or exercised too intensely.

Use the 15-minute rule. Always *start* your workout, no matter how energetic you're feeling, and go for 15 minutes. If you still feel like quitting after that, okay, do so without guilt. Your body may be telling you that it needs rest.

What if you wake up and think you're getting sick? I'd let your symptoms determine whether you should exercise. If you have fever or chest congestion, take the day off and perhaps see your doctor. (Seeing your doctor is a necessity if you feel chest congestion when you exercise: You could be at risk for infection in the heart, which can lead to a cardiomyopathy.) When your fever is gone and you feel better, ease back into exercise gradually.

Be patient. If you think you're getting a head cold, also use the 15-minute rule. Sometimes the symptoms will actually disappear while you exercise. If they worsen or you just don't feel good, stop. No guilt. You had 15 minutes of exercise, and you trusted your body. That's good.

Food Deprivation

Think about this kind of situation: You're planning a lunchtime workout near your house or office. But you didn't eat breakfast that morning and you are ravenously hungry. How likely are you to work out?

Does this sound familiar? "I do a lot of lunchtime workouts. If I don't eat breakfast, I simply won't work out at lunch. I love breakfast more than any meal, but I'm never hungry until 9 a.m., and by then I'm at work. So I have to eat at certain times whether or not I'm hungry if I'm going to have the energy when I need it. I can't use hunger as a signal. I have to eat something sustaining before I leave the house in the morning, and I have to plan to eat something after my lunch workout."

Skipping meals, along with a lack of exercise, is more than likely one of the largest causes of eating too much. What you want to do is maintain your energy by regularly eating healthy food. It's one of the simplest incentives for getting you moving and staying active.

Sleep Deprivation

We are a culture that brags about how little sleep we need. Well, maybe we can go without sleep for a while, but eventually we become sleep deprived.

Our sleep expert at Canyon Ranch, Phil Eichling, MD, suggests a simple measure to assess whether you have sleep deprivation. If you can fall asleep in a lecture—or, for that matter, while reading this book—you probably have sleep deprivation. But here's a more surprising test: If you need an alarm clock to wake you up every morning, it's *another* sign that you're sleep deprived!

A number of years ago, Phil said that his New Year's resolution was to wake up each morning without the prompting of an alarm clock. I tried it myself, just to see what would happen. The result? I have rarely used one since.

You might think you'd sleep 14 hours and miss half the day if your alarm didn't go off. Fear not. That doesn't happen if you're getting enough sleep every night. Most people will only sleep 7 to 8 hours per night. If I've had several hours or more of vigorous exercise, I might need 9 hours. But I usually get 8, and I no longer need midday naps.

If you do suffer from sleep deprivation, it might be caused by the choices you make. If you go to bed at 10 p.m. on weeknights, but choose to stay up until midnight on Friday, you change your rhythm. Sunday night, despite your early Monday schedule, you can't fall asleep, it's midnight, and you end up watching the biography of Wayne Newton on a channel you never even knew existed. And so, Monday, like many Americans, you wake up tired.

It's no wonder that the highest incidence of surgical accidents, errors made in factories, and motor vehicle accidents occurs on Mondays. After dragging yourself around all day, you look forward to going to sleep Monday at an earlier time, restoring your weekday schedule. Still, Monday was lost, so was your workout, and possibly your momentum in developing and keeping your exercise habit.

Common side effects of sleep deprivation include decreased cognitive function, lack of energy, high blood sugar, and weight gain. Lack of sleep may increase cortisol, that natural fight-or-flight hormone that surges through your system, providing energy in emergencies. Weight gain may be caused by such hormonal changes, but appetite changes with sleepiness may also account for the well-documented link to diabetes mellitus.

Choose to go to bed at a reasonable, regular hour and your health and exercise routine will benefit you in a host of ways.

Alcohol

Another cause of missed exercise due to sleep deprivation is alcohol consumption. Although alcohol is a depressant that helps you fall asleep, drinking is actually the worst thing you can do before going to bed.

Each drink is processed in your liver at about one drink per 2 hours, depending on your gender and size. (Large men tend to process alcohol faster than small women.) After the depressant effect wears off, there may be a surge of excitation. It's not necessarily enough to wake you up, but it's enough to prevent you from getting into deep, restorative sleep cycles. Allow enough time for your body to process alcohol before you go to bed—or limit yourself to only having alcohol with meals.

Although there are lots of studies showing that the antioxidants and resins in wine and beer are healthy, you can obtain the same benefits from fruits, vegetables, and exercise. At 120 to 150 calories per drink, alcohol may not be conducive to a light load on your joints or to the prevention of diabetes. It also increases the chances that you'll overeat and blow off your workout. If you imbibe, do so moderately, well before your bedtime, and after you exercise.

Caffeine

Caffeine is also a drug that activates your fight-or-flight response. It is processed in your liver and has a half-life of 3 to 7 hours. This means that when you're young, its concentration in your body diminishes by half in about 3 hours. By the time you are in your fifties, it's more likely to take about 7 hours for your liver to process half the caffeine that you consume.

Translation: If you have two cups of coffee at noon, by 7 p.m. there is an entire cup of coffee still stimulating your central nervous system. At 2 a.m. you still have half a cup of coffee in your system. And, at 9 a.m., when you have probably started on your next round of coffee, there is still one-quarter of a cup from the day before doing its "wake-up" job. (I love my morning coffee, but I don't have more than two cups after 9 a.m.)

Tea has caffeine, too, but unless it's steeped a long time it has less than coffee.

Coffee-flavored frozen yogurts and ice creams usually use real coffee and can also prevent sleep. Chocolate, for all of its antioxidant properties, also contains stimulants that are in the same family as caffeine. Too much at bedtime can result in a missed night's sleep and workout activities.

CREATING BACKUP STRATEGIES

Strategies for being fit must include contingency workouts. Some days you just won't have time for your regular routine. Don't think, "I don't have time for exercise today." Instead, consider how much exercise you *can* get. Be active in a different way. Go walking with friends. Or get out with some kids and toss the ball around.

A long time ago, I discovered that a shortened workout often whets your appetite for more. If you can't get in a half hour, do three 10-minute sessions. If you don't have time for your usual two sets of weights, perform one set. Or just do your squats or "core" exercises. Even if you don't get a chance to exercise more the same day, you'll come back the *next* day hungry for more.

Schedule and Track Your Workouts

If you have a meeting with your lawyer, doctor, accountant, or dentist, you make sure you get there at the appointed time. But a workout is often considered less important than other things, and you skip it for something that's "more important."

As we discussed earlier, the single best predictor of a long, healthy life is performing well on a cardiac stress test. (If you want to foretell the length and quality of your life, the cardiac stress test turns out to be more reliable than measurements of blood pressure, cholesterol level, or any other medical test.) People who do best on this test are those who recognize that their exercise appointment is paramount, and they keep that daily appointment.

What's the best way to do this? Well, you don't have to tell your client, "I can't meet you at 10 a.m., because it's my workout time." You simply say, "I can't meet you at 10 a.m., but how about 11 a.m.?" Exercise needs to go on your calendar. Write it in your appointment book, program your handheld, set the timer on your cell phone, and respect that appointment just as you would any other.

To keep track of your workout successes, hang that calendar in a place you will see it often, such as your bedroom, bathroom, or office wall. Every day that you work out, put up a stick-on star or write down, briefly, what you did. A visual reminder of your consistent success makes you feel fitter, and it validates your intention. You'll see at a glance which days you missed. The visual reminder will tell you to get back at it.

Consult with a Personal Trainer

If you can afford it, a personal trainer can boost your regular activity level. Knowing you have your appointment, and that you've already paid the trainer for the month, will certainly be an incentive. A good trainer can make workouts fun and challenging. He or she can also provide more variety than this book alone can give you.

Make sure you get a trainer who is certified with one of the major organizations. Canyon Ranch recommends trainers certified with:

O American College of Sports Medicine (www.acsm.org)

O National Strength and Conditioning Association (www.nsca-lift.org)

O National Academy of Sports Medicine (www.nasm.org)

O American Council on Exercise (www.acefitness.org)

A good trainer knows that no one should be pushed into strength-training sessions where the weight or resistance is constantly being increased all year-round. Instead, you'll be encouraged to gradually increase your strength for a period of 3 to 4 months, followed by a plateau period, during which you get used to the amount of weight.

During plateau periods, you work on maintaining strength and cardiovascular fitness or agility and balance. (You recover all of the joy!)

If you get a trainer who makes your workout seem like rocket science, and that just isn't your style, I'd advise you to find someone else. When workouts are too complicated, with many different sets and exercises, it's doubtful you'll receive the benefits I've presented here. (And it sure won't be much fun!) You want someone who keeps it simple. Your trainer should line up a maximum of 10 to 12 exercises, gradually increasing resistance.

Write down every repetition and resistance used. This is the only safe way to maximize your strength.

Change the Way You Think of Movement

There are more pleasurable ways to include movement in our lives than we realize. Do you like art? Go to museums and accumulate your 10,000 steps while enjoying the paintings and sculptures. Do you like history? Choose an historical place and plan a day visit, with walking and learning combined. What could be more enjoyable?

For years my family has chosen active vacations. One year we rented a condominium near a beautiful mountain town in Colorado. Every day we did something that was fun and active—mountain biking, hiking, horseback riding, kayaking.

When my wife and I go anywhere new, we love to explore on foot. As Gandhi said, "There is more to life than increasing its speed."

I believe that the slower the mode of transport, the richer the experience. Bicycling is better than riding in a car. Running, if your knees agree, may be even better. But the best, by far, is walking.

THE BEST PART OF YOUR LIFE

After finishing this book, I hope you feel inspired. You may sense your potential to live fully, every day of your life, for the rest of your life. . . .

Put on your shoes and go for a walk. Watch and appreciate this miracle called life, feel yourself right in the middle of it, and listen to your beautiful breath. What could be a sweeter experience?

INDEX

Boldface page references indicate illustrations (photographs). Underscored references indicate boxed text.

Ingrown toenails, 121

Injury

    flexibility relationship to, 30

    as impediment to exercise plans, 258

    law of resultant force, 20

    responding to, 20–21

Insulin, 13

Intensity, exercise

    Borg Perceived Exertion Scale, 9–10

    levels in exercise plan, 256

    moderate-intensity activities, xv

    predicted maximum heart rate, 8–9

Interdigital neuromas, 119–20

Intervertebral discs, 177

Inventory, before/after exercise feeling,
    252–55, _253_

Inversion sprain, 111, 113

ITBS. _See_ Iliotibial band syndrome (ITBS)

J

Joint. _See also specific joints_

    ball and socket, 153

    facet, 177

    hinge, 127

    hyperextended, 34

    pain, _34_

Joint mobilizations, _135_

Jumper's knee, 143

K

Knee

    anatomy

        general anatomy, 127, **128**, 129

        ligaments, **128**, 129–30

        menisci, **128**, 130

    cartilage damage in, _21_

    flexibility, 34

    hyperextended, 36, **36**, 155, _187_

hypomobile, _135_

injuries

    ACL (anterior cruciate ligament)
        rupture, 138, _139_

    bursitis, 143

    gender differences in risk, _139_

    iliotibial band syndrome (ITBS),
        144–47

    medical attention, need for, 137

    meniscus tear, 138–42

    muscle strains, 143

    overuse, 142–49

    runner's knee (patellofemoral
        syndrome), 147–49

    tendonitis, 143

    Ken's story, 132–34

    osteoarthritis, 127, 130–31, _131_

    pain, 125–26, _131_

    surgery, _129_, 130, _140_

    tibiofemoral rotation syndrome, 132,
        _135_, 135–37

Kneecap, 127, **128**, 130, 143, 147–48

Kyphosis, 93

L

Labrum, hip, 154–55, _156_

LaLanne, Jack (godfather of fitness), 57

Lateral shoulder raise in external rotation
    in plane of scapulae, 72, **72**

Latissimus dorsi muscle

    short and stiff, 22, 45, 225, 226

    underhand pulldown exercise, 68–69,
        68–69

Latissimus dorsi stretch, 45, **45**, 226

Latissimus dorsi test, 39, **39**, _202_

Lat pulldown, 226

Laughter, effect on pain, 237–40

Learning, exercise effect on, 5–6

Leg, length discrepancy in, 146–47

Leg press machine, 93, 98, 149, **149**, 171